Your Health at Work

Changing the world
of work for good

a TUC guide

Your Health
at Work

An indispensable guide to
physical and mental wellbeing

Becky Allen
Howard Fidderman

KoganPage

Publisher's note

Every possible effort has been made to ensure that the information contained in this book is accurate at the time of going to press, and the publishers and authors cannot accept responsibility for any errors or omissions, however caused. No responsibility for loss or damage occasioned to any person acting, or refraining from action, as a result of the material in this publication can be accepted by the editor, the publisher or the author.

First published in Great Britain and the United States in 2019 by Kogan Page Limited

2nd Floor, 45 Gee Street	c/o Martin P Hill Consulting	4737/23 Ansari Road
London	122 W 27th Street	Daryaganj
EC1V 3RS	New York, NY 10001	New Delhi 110002
United Kingdom	USA	India

© Trades Union Congress (TUC), Becky Allen and Howard Fidderman 2019

ISBN   978 0 7494 8150 6
E-ISBN   978 0 7494 8151 3

British Library Cataloguing-in-Publication Data

A CIP record for this book is available from the British Library.

Typeset by Integra Software Services Pvt. Ltd., Pondicherry
print production managed by Jellyfish
Printed and bound in Great Britain by Martins the Printers

Contents

Introduction

This book is about your health at work. It is written by experts in the field, and supported by the TUC and its member unions, who fought for many of the health rights that workers enjoy today. Unions achieve change by representing you collectively at work.

Twenty years ago, this book would have focused mainly on specific diseases and disorders that were caused or made worse by your work. It would have looked at musculoskeletal disorders and occupational diseases such as cancer, as well as the then emerging issue of stress. And it would have dealt with a health and safety system in which the main players were the Health and Safety Executive (HSE) and local authorities (which together inspect and enforce health and safety legislation at your workplaces), trade unions and some large employers and employers' organizations. While all these elements remain relevant and important, safeguarding your health at work is today bound up in wider considerations and influences.

Despite the huge changes in the ways that many of us work, and the evidence we have from research about how to reduce the impact of work on health, some 1.3 million people in Britain suffer from illnesses caused – or made worse – by work (which amounts to 25.7 million workdays lost each year). This toll includes 8,000 deaths a year from occupational cancers – itself a conservative estimate – and 13,500 new cancer registrations. Aside from the physical and mental suffering endured by workers and their families, work-related illness also has a massive impact on the economy. New cases of work-related illness cost individuals, employers and the government around £9.7 billion in 2016/17, over half of which is borne by individuals.[1]

Most work-related illness is easily preventable. Trade unions have worked tirelessly over many years to make workplaces healthier. We have legislation in the UK – the Health and Safety at Work Act from 1974 and dozens of sets of regulations, many of which implement European law – designed to prevent you and your colleagues from being made ill by work. And a 2016 guideline from the Sentencing Council has meant that employers are increasingly receiving fines that match their crimes, with the total amount of fines imposed almost trebling in the first full year in which the guideline was in force, even though the number of prosecutions decreased.[2]

Today, your health at work encompasses broader issues and reflects major changes in the UK's population, economy and government and societal priorities. Politically, we live in a de-regulatory climate in which health and safety is often depicted as a 'burden on business' – until, that is, something goes terribly wrong. And with so much of our health at work legislation emanating from the EU, these protections and rights face an uncertain and possibly precarious future. Crosscutting themes recur throughout the book, as well as being covered in specific chapters on the ageing workforce, migrant workers, young workers and apprentices, new ways of working, disability and mental health issues. Together, all of these factors are having a major impact on your health at work.

The UK population – and its workforce – is ageing. We explain why this is happening and how it affects your health at work. Successive governments – regardless of political persuasion – have introduced policies that encourage people to work but, in the bad cases, force people to work or find work when not completely healthy. The emphasis for the state is now on what you can do rather than what you cannot do. Work should be good for you, but you need to ensure that it works for you. The economy is also changing, so we look at the rise of the gig economy and zero-hours contracts and the health risks these present. And we look at how social and political changes are expanding what we mean by health at work.

These changes are arguably most apparent in mental health. Recent years have seen a marked shift in attitudes to mental health in schools, communities and workplaces. Mental illness is the single largest cause of disability in the UK. It affects one in four of us and costs the economy around £100 billion a year – roughly the cost of the entire NHS. There are close links between mental and physical health, with conditions that were previously treated separately increasingly approached as a whole – for example, musculoskeletal disorders and stress-related conditions. If you have a severe, long-term mental illness, you are likely to die 10–20 years earlier than other people, making this a huge source of health inequality.[3] The NHS spends only 13% of its budget on mental health services, although it is working to redress this imbalance in spending, services and care.[4]

Mental health is not only about healthcare; it is a workplace issue. Together with musculoskeletal disorders and occupational lung diseases, mental health is one of the HSE's three strategic health priorities.[5] Separately, in 2017, the Prime Minister asked Lord Dennis Stevenson, a mental health campaigner, and Paul Farmer, CEO of Mind, to conduct an independent review of how employers can facilitate mental health support for employees with mental health problems. According to their report, *Thriving at work*,[6] the UK is facing a mental health challenge at work that is much larger than they had thought. Their vision is that in 10 years' time: employees in all types of employment will have 'good work'; that all organizations, large and small, will have the tools and awareness to address and prevent mental ill health caused or made worse by work; and that all of us will have the information and confidence to look after our own mental health and the mental health of those around us. And in October 2017, the Prime Minister confirmed that NHS England and the Civil Service – two of the country's largest employers – would implement the report's recommendations.

This book reflects these and other changes, including the renewed focus on how workplaces can support healthier lifestyles, the growing awareness of the importance of sleep, and breaking the taboo surrounding menopause and suicide so that we can create supportive working environments where people feel able to talk about difficult issues. It also includes a diverse range of voices, including third sector organizations such as Samaritans, Macmillan Cancer Support and Business in the Community, which are helping to redefine health at work and are providing vital information, advice and support.

We think that all these changes make this book particularly timely. Our aim is to look at how the changes are affecting your health at work and to give you – in an accessible and comprehensive way – a picture of the legal landscape, the latest research, examples of best practice and new case studies. We also indicate the best sources of further help, if you need any. Nearly all of this help is free.

While it remains your employer's legal duty to protect your health and safety at work, we believe that everyone should be informed, involved and equipped to help secure their health at work and, if things go wrong, know what to do and where to seek help. And while this book is aimed at individual workers, we believe unequivocally that, to make workplaces healthier, we need collective action. That is where unions come in. If you do one thing after reading this, make it joining a trade union.

Notes

1 www.hse.gov.uk/statistics/cost.htm

2 HSE (2018) *Health and safety at work. Summary statistics for Great Britain 2017.* www.hse.gov.uk/statistics/overall/hssh1617.pdf

3 Public Health England (2018) *Wellbeing and Mental Health: Applying all our health.* Available from www.gov.uk/government/publications/wellbeing-in-mental-health-applying-all-our-health/wellbeing-in-mental-health-applying-all-our-health

4 Statistic from House of Commons Library (2017) 'Mental health policy in England', researchbriefings.files.parliament.uk/documents/CBP-7547/CBP-7547.pdf

5 HSE (2016) *Health and Work strategy.* www.hse.gov.uk/aboutus/strategiesandplans/health-and-work-strategy/health-and-work-strategy.pdf

6 Farmer P, Stevenson D (2017) *Thriving at work: The Stevenson/Farmer review of mental health and employers.* bit.ly/2hd3ApX

Chapter 1
Safeguarding mental health

At any one time, one in six adults in the UK is experiencing a mental health condition, according to the Department of Health.[1] Many of these individuals will also be workers, but while most common problems are successfully treated, 300,000 people with a long-term mental health problem still lose their job every year. In this chapter, we look at what you and your employer can do to secure good mental health and how to help you and your colleagues if you are suffering mental ill health. Helping people with mental health issues to find and stay in work brings benefits to the individual worker, the employer and the economy, as will be explained in more detail later.

Mental health can be a wide-ranging and even vague concept, with the Health and Safety Executive (HSE) defining it as 'how we think, feel and behave'. Mental ill health ranges from specific conditions to collections of less precise symptoms. The mental health charity, MIND, lists more than 30 types of mental health problems, including bipolar disorder,[2] anxiety and panic attacks, eating disorders, loneliness, obsessive-compulsive disorder, phobias, sleep problems, stress and suicidal feelings. All in all, one in four people in the UK will have a mental health problem at some point in their lives.[3]

Thirty years ago, most workers with mental health issues did not expect to receive significant help from their employer beyond, in the more enlightened or benevolent cases, tolerance and some time off work. For the government and the bodies that enforce health and safety at work – the HSE and local authorities – the emphasis had traditionally been on safety with consideration of health matters mostly addressing physical health. The focus has been shifting, however; not least because of pressure from trade unions, mental health campaigners and health professionals. The result is that the HSE and government are encouraging employers to address the relationship between the workplace and mental ill health. In particular they are looking to prevent work-related matters causing or exacerbating a mental health condition, help individuals to cope with a condition, and persuade employers and workers that good work and good mental health go hand in hand.

The most significant change at policy and regulatory level came with the HSE's development of the stress management standards, which it first published in 2004 (see chapter 2). These have formed the basis for the approach of many employers that have tried to address stress. Mental health, however, is far wider an issue than stress alone and the government is increasingly expecting employers to address mental health, even if it has failed to back its pronouncements with enough resources.

In 2017, a major independent review of ways to facilitate good mental health and to support workers with mental health problems or poor wellbeing to remain in work[4] recommended a raft of measures that should be taken by employers, the NHS, the HSE, local authorities, the government and others to improve mental health at work. The government accepted the recommendations in January 2018, but it will need to redress the past cuts in budgets and reductions in the provision of some services if workers are to benefit from some of the commitments.

The law

The legislation governing mental health at work is essentially that which governs physical health and safety. At its core is the

Health and Safety at Work Act 1974, which requires employers to ensure the safety and health (including mental health) of employees. Similarly, the Management of Health and Safety at Work Regulations 1999 (MHSW) apply to mental health as they do to physical health and safety. They require employers to carry out a risk assessment and then to make arrangements for the planning, organization, control, monitoring and review of the preventive and protective measures that they identify as needed.

A schedule to the MHSW Regulations sets out nine general principles of prevention, starting with avoiding risks in the first place. Where this is not possible, three of the principles are potentially of particular significance for mental health:

- 'adapting the work to the individual, especially as regards the design of workplaces, the choice of work equipment and the choice of working and production methods, with a view, in particular, to alleviating monotonous work and work at a predetermined work-rate and to reducing their effect on health';

- 'developing a coherent overall prevention policy which covers technology, organisation of work, working conditions, social relationships and the influence of factors relating to the working environment'; and

- 'giving collective protective measures priority over individual protective measures'.[5]

The Working Time Regulations 1998 set out requirements relating to maximum weekly working hours, the duration of night work, health assessment for night work, patterns of work, daily rest, weekly rest periods, rest breaks, annual leave and shift work (see chapters 9 and 10). Although the Regulations refer to health generally (rather than mental or physical health), the provisions are significant for mental health.

Access to work

The Equality Act 2010 protects individuals with disabilities against discrimination or detriment as a result of their disability. Disability under the Act is a physical or mental impairment that 'has a substantial and long-term adverse effect' (12 months in practice) on the person's ability to carry out normal day-to-day activities. Crucially, your employer must make reasonable adjustments to any elements of your job that place you at a substantial disadvantage compared to persons who are not disabled. We look in detail at reasonable adjustments in chapter 7.

Where the help that you need to start, remain in, or return to work is not covered by your employer's legal duty to make reasonable adjustments, you can apply to the government's Access to Work scheme.[6] This covers individuals who are disabled or have a mental or physical health condition that affects their work. The scheme applies to paid work (including self-employment, apprenticeships, work trials, work experience and internships). It can offer you support, based on your needs, and can include a grant to help cover the costs of a support service if you have a mental health condition (which could include counselling or job coaching), a support worker or job coach, or help getting to and from work (including taxi fares to work or a support worker if you cannot use public transport).

After you have applied, an Access to Work adviser will contact you to discuss possible assistance. The adviser may also contact your employer but will only do so after first having spoken to you. An assessor may visit your workplace to determine your needs.

Remploy

Remploy offers a free Workplace Mental Health Support Service[7] for employees who are suffering depression, anxiety, stress or other mental health issues that have caused absence or problems remaining in work. Remploy advises that the service, which is funded by the Department for Work and Pensions, has helped 10,000 workers, with 93% of users retaining their employment after six months. Its specialist advisers offer:

- tailored work-focused mental health support for six months;
- coping strategies;
- a support plan to keep individuals in work or help them return to work;
- ideas for workplace adjustments to help individuals fulfil their roles; and
- practical advice to support individuals with a mental health condition.

Remploy offers a similar service for apprentices[8] as well as advice for employers, resources, 'Champion networks' and mental health training.[9]

The core mental health standards

The 2017 Stevenson-Farmer independent review of mental health and work set out six core mental health standards. Among these are that your employer should:

- implement, and communicate to the workforce, a mental health at work plan that includes the support on offer, including offers of reasonable adjustment, at recruitment and at regular intervals thereafter;
- develop mental health awareness among you and your colleagues;
- provide you with good working conditions and ensure you have a healthy work life balance and opportunities to develop; and

- ensure you speak regularly with your line manager or supervisor. One of the problems for people with mental health problems is 'speaking out'. The review found that four in five employers had no employees disclosing a mental health condition but one in two employees will not discuss mental health issues with their line manager.

If you work in the public sector or for a private sector company with more than 500 employees, the review recommended your employer should also deliver four enhanced mental health standards, which include a 'leadership commitment' and a nominated lead at board or senior level, as well as ensuring there is tailored in-house mental health support and signposting to clinical help that includes occupational health services or employee assistance programmes (EAPs) paid for by the employer as well as NHS services.

If your employer is reluctant to address mental health issues, it is worth making sure it knows that it should be able to meet the standards at little or no cost in the first place, and that studies of individual organizations and academic research show that interventions secure a positive return on investment. The 2017 independent government-commissioned review estimated the overall annual cost of mental illness to the economy as a whole at between £74 billion and £99 billion. Of this, employers bear £33–42 billion, over half of which is attributable to presenteeism, (where workers with poor mental health are present at work but are less productive).[10] At some point in the future, your employer will be able to access a mental health online information portal recommended by the review that will help implement the standards. In the meantime, there are numerous other sources of advice and information, some of which are covered in this chapter and the next chapter on stress. Encourage your employer too to arrange for mental health at work training (only one in four managers have received such training).

Mental Health First Aiders

In the past decade, almost 200,000 Mental Health First Aiders (MHFAs)[11] have been trained in the UK. In 2017, the Conservative Party's General Election manifesto promised that it would amend health and safety legislation 'so that employers provide appropriate first aid training and needs-assessment for mental health, as they currently do for risks to physical health'.[12] Although the government has not published any legislative proposals, it did announce funding of £15 million for a programme to train one million people in basic mental health 'first aid' skills.

Once trained, people should be better placed to notice and help a person who may have a mental health issue, including by signposting them to support services.

Although there is no conclusive evidence of the impact at work of MHFAs, the trained MHFAs are undoubtedly better informed and more aware of mental health issues and there are reports of how they have helped individuals with problems. Remember, however, that the clue is in the title: MHFAs are a first aid responder when things have gone wrong. They are not a solution and they are certainly not an alternative to your employer managing the issue appropriately through preventive and anti-discriminatory policies, proper procedures and access to occupational health services.[13]

What to do

The box on page 13 sets out some indicators of poor mental health. Should some of these indicators apply to you, the sooner you act, the better. Unfortunately, some workers still feel embarrassed if they have a mental health problem, or fear suffering detriment or discrimination as a result of talking about mental health issues at work. The most important first step is to see your

GP, who may refer you for specialist help, including counselling. MIND offers advice and factsheets on the main mental health conditions.[14] At work, talk to colleagues and your union or staff representative. You should also talk to your line manager or supervisor and, depending on the size of the organization for which you work, the HR and occupational health departments. Your representative will also be able to help you take the matter forward with your employer. There are many organizations that might offer advice; see for example Mindful Employer, an NHS initiative that started in southwest England but now operates nationwide.[15]

If you have been off work, agree a written plan for return with your manager before you return. You may need a phased return, which can involve reduced hours, days or workload. Your employer may be required to make reasonable adjustments under the Equality Act 2010 to facilitate your return.

Mental ill health indicators

Specific mental health conditions will often have particular symptoms. The symptoms listed below are commonly associated with mental ill health, but they may also be symptomatic of another condition. It would be worth consulting your GP if you be experiencing some of the symptoms below:

- withdrawal from social situations and friends, family and colleagues;
- a marked drop in functioning or difficulty performing familiar tasks;
- difficulties in concentrating or remembering;
- increased sensitivity to sights, sounds and smells or touch;
- a lack of desire to participate in activities;

- feeling disconnected from yourself or your surroundings;
- thinking that is not logical;
- nervousness;
- unusual or uncharacteristic behaviour;
- changes in sleep patterns;
- changes in appetite;
- rapid mood changes and outbursts of anger;
- mood changes over several weeks;
- your behaviour is having a negative impact on other people;
- thoughts of suicide;
- you often feel tired at work;
- outbursts of anger.

Wellness Action Plans

Developed by Mary Ellen Copeland in 1997, WRAP (Wellness Recovery Action Plan) is an evidence-based system used worldwide by people to manage their mental health. Inspired by this system, Mind has developed a Wellness Action Plan[16] (WAP) to help employees 'support their own mental health by reflecting on the causes of stress and poor mental health, and by taking ownership of practical steps to help address these triggers'.

Mind believes that all workers should be offered a WAP, regardless of whether they are suffering from mental health problems, because planning in advance ensures that all workers receive the support they need, when they need it. It also 'facilitates open dialogue' between employees and managers. Mind suggests that employees draft the WAP, with support from a health professional where appropriate, and then discuss and agree it with the manager.

Mind offers a template for a WAP (see box) and advises that it should cover:

- actions and behaviours that support the employee's mental wellbeing;

- symptoms, early warning signs and triggers for poor mental health or stress;

- potential impact of poor mental health or a mental health problem on the employee's performance;

- the support employees need from their line manager;

- positive steps for the employees to take if they are experiencing stress or poor mental health; and

- an agreed time to review the efficacy of the support measures.

Mind's Wellness Action Plan template

1 What helps you stay mentally healthy at work? (For example, taking a lunch break, keeping a to-do list.)

2 What can your manager do to support you to stay mentally healthy at work? (For example, regular feedback and supervision, explaining wider developments in the organization.)

3 Are there any situations at work that can trigger poor mental health for you? (For example, conflict at work, organizational change, something not going to plan.)

4 How might stress/poor mental health difficulties impact on your work? (For example, find it difficult to make decisions, hard to prioritize work tasks.)

5 Are there any early warning signs that we might notice when you are starting to feel stressed/ mentally unwell? (For example, changes in normal working patterns, withdrawing from colleagues.)

6 What support could be put in place to minimize triggers or to support you to manage symptoms? (For example, extra catch-up time with line manager.)

7 If we notice early warning signs that you are feeling stressed or unwell, what should we do? (For example, talk to me discreetly about it, contact someone that I have asked to be contacted.) Please include contact names and numbers if you would like your line manager to get in touch with someone if you become unwell.

8 What steps can you take if you start to feel unwell at work? (For example, take a break from your desk and go for a short walk, ask your line manager for support.)

Helping yourself

Although your employer is under a duty to ensure your mental health at work and is therefore responsible for assessing the risks you face and for implementing measures to safeguard your wellbeing, there is a great deal of advice available about how you can give yourself the best chance of mental health and well-being. It is important to remember, however, that not all the advice is supported by robust or conclusive evidence and that different things may work for different people. In the section below, we draw on advice from sources that include Mind and the Mental Health Foundation[17] (mental health charities), the New Economics Foundation (a think tank),[18] the NHS[19] and the government.

Managing time

- Make sure you have a good balance between your work and non-work life, with working long hours and overtime the exception and not the rule. Keep clear boundaries between work and home. If you do have to take work home, or work from home, a specific area for work can help maintain physical and mental separation.

- Take a break. This can range from as little as five minutes away from your desk, to a weekend break. Plan your leave so that you have something to look forward to. Try to avoid checking into work through email or texts when you are on a break.

- Use your lunch break. You could initiate or join a group activity (such as a game or a walk), or take up a challenge such as running and training with colleagues.

- Use the work commute to set aside some time for yourself so that you can read or listen to a podcast or music. Listening to music can also take your mind off work and reduce anxiety, block out noise and eliminate distractions.

Physical

- Regular physical activity can help to reduce depression and anxiety, boost self-esteem and may decrease the pace of cognitive decline as you age. The activity need not be intense: you do not have to run a marathon or go to the gym; walking or a class will suffice. Slower paced exercise such as walking may even encourage social interaction. Simple steps can include walking to work, up stairs (rather than using a lift), and going over to a colleague's desk rather than contacting them by phone or email.

Regular exercise – aim for 30 minutes a day – can help you concentrate, sleep, and look and feel better.

- Eat properly. Although it can be harder to eat well at work, many workplaces will have healthy lunch options, or you can bring lunch from home. Try too to eat lunch away from your desk.

Positive mental habits

- Learning throughout life enhances self-esteem and can encourage social interaction. Achieving learning goals is linked to improved wellbeing. Tips include signing up for a class, reading the news, setting up a book club, or researching something of interest.

- Do something you are good at and enjoy, for example a hobby, gardening, a book club or cycling.

- Consider 'mindfulness', which is proving increasingly popular as a technique for coping with some mental health issues, although it attracts controversy. The National Institute for Health and Care Excellence (NICE), for example, recommends mindfulness as a prevention technique for people who have had three or more bouts of depression. NHS Choices[20] describes mindfulness as 'knowing directly what is going on inside and outside of ourselves, moment by moment. It involves reconnecting with your body and being aware of your thoughts and feelings.' Enjoy the moment, too, and take notice of how your colleagues are feeling. You are, after all, not alone as, statistically, one in four of your colleagues is also likely to be suffering from a mental health issue.

Other people

- Try to connect with other people. Social relationships both help promote wellbeing and prevent mental ill health. You could talk to, and not email, a colleague, speak to someone new, or share a journey to or from work with a colleague.

- Participation in social and community life and helping others brings benefits. An act of kindness once a week for six weeks, according to Mind, 'is associated with an increase in wellbeing'. Some companies grant paid time off to staff to participate in community or voluntary work.

- Take particular care of your mental health if you also have caring responsibilities for a child, parent or friend. While work can provide a respite for carers, it is also important that it takes account of your situation away from work.

- Talk about your feelings with someone with whom you feel comfortable and who will be supportive. If it is difficult to do this at work, discuss work pressures with a partner, friend or family member.

- A supportive team at work is important to your mental health at work. There will sometimes be tensions, both personal and work-related, and it is important to know how to look after yourself and address problems. It can be helpful to find a mentor or a small group of trusted colleagues to help you navigate difficulties.

- Ask for help. Your employer may use an employee assistance programme and an internal or external occupational health service. These will be free for you to use and confidential. Your GP may refer you to a counsellor, but this is not always free, particularly if you are unable to wait.

CASE STUDY Mates in Mind

Mates in Mind[21] is an initiative that aims to improve mental health awareness and education, and to prevent suicide, among construction workers. The initiative was established by the Health in Construction Leadership Group, with the support of the British Safety Council. Mental Health First Aid England, Mind and Samaritans are core partners.

The group encourages construction employers to implement a mental health programme that 'drives a culture of speaking up' and helps safeguard the mental health of the workforce. Mates in Mind was launched in January 2017 and, following a pilot among six companies in the first half of 2017, aims to reach 75% of the construction workforce by 2025. Some construction companies have said that participation will be a requirement for their contractors.

The services will be provided through partners. The Mates in Mind website offers contacts for workers who need help, including Samaritans, Construction Industry Helpline, Mind Info-line and Remploy. It encourages workers to talk to colleagues to see whether they have any problems, and provides advice on healthy working and living.

Mates in Mind offers health promotional materials and a two-day mental health first aid course after which individuals become 'Mates in Mind workplace champions'. It also provides a 45-minute induction course and a 3.5-hour course for forepersons, supervisors and managers.

Mates In Mind claims that working patterns and demands are at particular risk in the industry. Moreover, 350,000 construction workers may be suffering from depression, anxiety or stress at any one time and they are more likely to be at risk of mental ill health than other workers. The number of suicides is 10 times as high as the number of fatal injuries in the industry.

Notes

1 Department of Health (2012) *Advice for employers on workplace adjustments for mental health conditions.* www.nhshealthatwork. co.uk/images/library/files/government%20policy/Mental_Health_ Adjustments_Guidance_May_2012.pdf

2 www.bipolaruk.org/pages/search.aspx?q=workplace

3 www.hse.gov.uk/stress/mental-health.htm

4 Farmer P, Stevenson D (2017) *Thriving at work. The Stevenson/ Farmer review of mental health and employers.* bit.ly/2hd3ApX

5 www.legislation.gov.uk/uksi/1999/3242/schedule/1/made

6 www.gov.uk/access-to-work

7 www.remploy.co.uk/employers/mental-health-and-wellbeing/ workplace-mental-health-support-service-employers

8 Remploy Apprentices Service: 0300 456 8210 or apprentices@ remploy.co.uk. Details and information: www.remploy.co.uk/ employers/mental-health-and-wellbeing/supporting-apprentices- service

9 www.remploy.co.uk/employers/mental-health-and-wellbeing

10 Farmer P, Stevenson D, *Thriving at work.* See also the cost analysis undertaken for the review by Deloitte: www.deloitte. co.uk/MentalHealthReview

11 MHFA England: mhfaengland.org

12 *Forward, together. Our plan for a stronger Britain and a prosperous future. The Conservative and Unionist Party manifesto 2017.* bit.ly/2ruEdCy

13 For details and an appraisal, see Robertson H, 'Is mental health first aid the answer? Depends on the questions', *Hazards magazine*, number 141, 2018. www.hazards.org/stress/ mentalhealth.htm

14 www.mind.org.uk/information-support/types-of-mental-health- problems

15 www.mindfulemployer.net/employees

16 Mind, *Guide to Wellness Action Plans*. www.mind.org.uk/
media/1593680/guide-to-waps.pdf

17 Mental Health Foundation: www.mentalhealth.org.uk/our-work/
mental-health-workplace

18 www.mentalhealth.org.uk/publications/how-support-mental-
health-work

19 www.nhs.uk/conditions/stress-anxiety-depression/improve-
mental-wellbeing

20 www.nhs.uk/conditions/stress-anxiety-depression/mindfulness

21 *Mates in Mind*: bit.ly/2n7Y2NB

Chapter 2
Tackling stress

Stress is an adverse reaction to excessive pressures or demands in your work life, home life or both. Prolonged periods of stress can adversely affect the way you feel, your behaviour and your health. At work, it is vital that your employer addresses stress by tackling the root causes of any stress that your work is causing or exacerbating. Too many employers instead focus on stress management programmes and techniques to help stressed workers cope with the symptoms of stress. Coping techniques have their place but they are not an alternative to addressing how you work.

As we note in the previous chapter, one in four people in the UK will have a mental health problem at some point in their lives, the most common of which are anxiety and depression. The HSE (Health and Safety Executive) advises that the key differences between common mental health problems and stress 'are their cause and the way they are treated'.[1] They often share symptoms, however, and work-related stress can aggravate and become entangled with an existing mental health problem. They can also exist independently – people can experience work-related stress and physical changes such as high blood pressure, without having anxiety and depression. They can also have anxiety and depression without stress.

To complicate matters further, the HSE groups stress, depression and anxiety as a single entity, estimating that they accounted for 40% (526,000) of all new and existing self-reported work-related ill health cases in 2016/17 and 49% (12.5 million) of working days lost from ill health. New cases amounted to 236,000 of the 526,000 cases.[2] The estimated cost of work-related stress, depression and anxiety is £5.2 billion to industry, individuals and the government.[3] Moreover, the TUC's most recent biennial survey of safety representatives found that stress 'stands out more than ever as the chief health and safety concern, identified as a top-five hazard by 70% of safety representatives in the survey'.[4]

Raised rates of stress can be found in any job, but the three sectors with rates of stress that are above the all industry average are human health and social work, public administration and defence, and education.[5] The main cause of these cases, according to the HSE, was workload (44%), followed by a lack of support (14%), violence, threats or bullying (13%) and changes at work (8%).[6] This will only be part of the story as workers are facing increasing job insecurity through zero-hours contracts, temporary contracts and low pay.

A simple approach to stress at work

Your employer has a general duty under the HSW Act 1974 to look after your health and ensure your safety at work. It also has a duty to carry out and implement the findings of a risk assessment under the Management of Health and Safety at Work Regulations 1999. Both of these duties apply to work-related stress. It is, however, worth reminding your employer of the benefits of addressing stress, beyond its legal duty and the avoidance of litigation. These include improvements in employee happiness, commitment to work, performance, productivity and attendance. Tackling stress can also improve the quality of working life, the management of change, employee relationships, staff retention rates, accident rates, customer satisfaction, and an organization's reputation.

A good approach would be for your employer to follow the HSE's guidance on stress. This involves the same five-step approach to risk assessment as for any other risk and the use of the HSE's six stress Management Standards.[7] Acas offers guidance that follows the standards closely.[8] Although your employer does not have to use the standards, it must use an equivalent approach. The HSE has produced a workbook for the standards, which makes it clear that 'The Management Standards approach relies on senior management commitment and worker involvement throughout the process.' You or your colleagues should therefore be involved in any stress working groups or equivalent.

The standards cover the six key areas of work design that, if not properly managed, are associated with poor health, lower productivity and increased accident and sickness absence rates. Although the standards are aimed at employers,[9] they are of significant value to workers as they highlight the issues that you should consider. Unusually for HSE guidance, each of the standards explicitly requires that employees 'indicate' to the employer that their situation accords with many of the elements of the standard. Each standard also requires the presence of local systems for responding to any concerns that you might have.

The six standards

The first standard covers work demands, which includes issues such as workload, work patterns and the work environment. The standard requires you to indicate that you are able to cope with the demands of your job. You should expect your employers to provide you with demands that are achievable within your agreed hours of work and appropriate to your skills, abilities and capabilities.

The second standard relates to control and how much say you have over how you work. Where possible, you should have control over the pace of your work. You should be consulted over your work patterns and over when breaks can be taken. Control also means that you are encouraged to use your skills and initiative to do your work and to develop new skills.

The third standard requires that you receive adequate information and support from your organization, line managers and colleagues. Support includes encouragement, sponsorship and resources. There should be systems in place to enable and encourage employees to support their colleagues and managers to support their staff. The standard also requires you to be aware of the support and resources that are available for you to do your job, and how and when to access them. You should also receive regular and constructive feedback on your work.

The fourth standard involves promoting positive working and behaviours to avoid conflict and ensure fairness. You must not be subject to unacceptable behaviours, for example bullying. Where behaviour is unacceptable, the organization should have agreed policies and procedures to prevent or resolve the behaviour, and enable and encourage you to report it and managers to deal with it.

The fifth standard requires that you understand your role and responsibilities within the organization and that your employer ensures that you do not have conflicting roles. Your employer needs to ensure that, as far as possible, the requirements that it places upon you are clear and compatible and that you have the information you need to understand your role and responsibilities.

The sixth standard relates to how organizational change is managed and communicated. You should be provided with timely information to enable you to understand the reasons for proposed changes, be consulted adequately and have the opportunity to influence proposals and be aware of the timetable. You should be aware of the probable impact of any changes to your job, receive training to support any changes and have access to support during changes.

Finally, to return to the point with which we started this chapter, the HSE emphasizes that the focus should be 'on prevention and on managing the root causes of work-related stress, rather than trying to deal with problems only after they occur and people are suffering from exposure to excessive pressure'. [10] It also reminds employers: 'When assessing the risks to which your employees may be exposed it is important to focus on organisational level issues that have the potential to impact on groups and large numbers of employees, rather than individual employees.' [11]

Relaunching and refreshing the standards

Despite widespread support from trade unions, employers and mental health professionals, the stress Management Standards have not enjoyed a large take-up, particularly by smaller firms. This led the HSE to re-launch the standards in March 2017. The standards were criticized in late 2017, however, by an independent review of mental health and work [12] commissioned by the Prime Minister, Theresa May, and carried out by Paul Farmer, the CEO of Mind, and Lord Dennis Stevenson, a mental health campaigner.

This review found that while the standards were a 'first step', they could potentially encourage employers to take a narrow approach because employees with mental health problems can present or face particular risks at work regardless of whether or not their condition was caused by work. The government accepted the review's recommendations and, as a result, the HSE will by April 2019 incorporate a 'more holistic approach' to show how its standards can help employers deliver key parts of the review's mental health core standards, which are more wide-ranging. The HSE will also revise its stress management guidance to raise employers' awareness of their duty to assess and manage work-related mental ill health and look to 'increase the focus on workplace mental health and safety during its inspections'. From an employee point of view, however, any changes the HSE might make does not undermine the importance of the current standards to the workplace.

Is there a problem at your workplace?

To help inform its approach to stress, your employer will look at sickness absence, productivity and turnover records but should also seek your views:

- Performance appraisals allow you to discuss how you are coping with your workload, discuss stressors and reasonable adjustments that might help you.

- You can raise issues and stressors in team meetings, which might also reveal similar and different stressors among your colleagues.

- Ensure that stress or stress-related issues is on the agenda of meetings, particularly where holiday and peak work demands are planned.

- You can ask your employer to use the HSE Management Standards indicator tool or an equivalent survey.[13] The HSE's tool asks 35 questions of employees across the six standards. It is important, however, not to take the results at face value as they may be skewed by a particularly good (or bad) department. The HSE notes that while self-reporting surveys are often questioned, 'evidence suggests that individual perceptions play an important role in predicting stress-related ill health', which means that 'gathering the opinions of employees can be a useful indicator of the health of your organization'.

The HSE suggests ten groups of questions where 'yes' answers might indicate that the work includes work-related stressors.[14] Although they are aimed at the employer, we have 'tweaked' them so that you can easily ask them of yourself and your colleagues (see table 2.1).

It is important that your employer discusses with you what it has found, not least because it might be that the highest-scoring stressors are not the most important on the ground. You should encourage your employer to use focus groups to discuss and develop solutions; the HSE advises that the optimum size of such a group is between six and ten people.

TABLE 2.1 Questions to ask yourself

		Yes	No
1	Is your role vocational (for example a nurse or teacher)?		
2	Does your role involve dealing with customers, or service users? If so, do the customers' relatives have direct access to you? Do you face a threat of third-party violence? Does a large proportion of your role involve dealing with complaints?		
3	Is your work reactive, ie does your workload depend on customers and their individual issues?		
4	Are you issued with equipment that makes you contactable out of normal working hours?		
5	Do your customers think they have a right to the service, benefit or product with which you are dealing, and will they be worse off if they do not receive it? Is your intervention likely to be unwelcome?		
6	Are changes imposed on your work by your head office or by outside regional or national bodies or authorities?		
7	Is your organization subject to periodic external scrutiny or inspection?		
8	Does the organization have strictly imposed rules on sickness absence and/or performance and are pay rises linked to performance or attendance?		
9	Does the organization have a 'macho' approach to stress or mental ill health?		
10	Has your organization recently been subject to changes that have: increased your workload; reduced the size of the workforce but not the amount of work; resulted in areas being understaffed; or changed the type or rate of your work?		
	Total		

Stress indicators and ill-health conditions

There is a wide range of potential signs of stress and of ill-health conditions that may arise in workers. The list below is drawn from bodies such as the HSE, TUC and the NHS. It is important to remember that people experience the effects of stress in different ways and, just because you exhibit some symptoms, it does not mean that you are suffering from stress. If the indicators or conditions persist, you should visit your GP. Make sure you discuss with your GP the type of work that you do and any impact you believe your work might be having. The indicators are broadly grouped into the way you act and feel, and medical conditions.

You may find yourself:

- taking more time off work;
- arriving for work later;
- behaving differently or more aggressively;
- interacting with your colleagues in a different way;
- more prone to mistakes or accidents;
- unable to delegate tasks;
- unable to focus;
- eating more or less than usual;
- smoking or drinking more than usual or taking drugs; and
- experiencing difficulty sleeping.

You may feel:

- nervous or twitchy;
- negative or lacking motivation, commitment and confidence;

- indecisive;
- isolated;
- unable to concentrate;
- moody (with mood swings); and
- withdrawn, isolated or difficult to contact.

Ill-health conditions can include:

- chronic anxiety, depression, mental breakdown and suicide;
- heart disease and attack, stroke and hypertension (high blood pressure);
- back pain and other musculoskeletal disorders;
- headaches and sweats;
- gastrointestinal disturbances, digestion problems, diarrhoea, vomiting and stomach ulcers;
- chronic dermatitis and other skin conditions;
- lowered resistance to infections;
- chronic asthma; and
- (possible) increased risk of cancer.

What you can do

If you think you are suffering from stress, you should talk to your GP, who may provide you with advice, refer you to a mental health specialist or for counselling, or prescribe medication. Although you may not want to talk about stress at work, possibly because of embarrassment or fear of stigma or suffering detriment, you should speak with someone at work with whom you feel comfortable. Ideally, this should be your union steward or union health and safety representative or, if your workplace does not have a recognized union, an employee representative or a colleague. Talk to your line or team manager. If you are not comfortable doing this – and it may be that the stressor involves your manager or a colleague – you may prefer to talk to the HR department. Your employer may have an in-house or external occupational health service or access to an employee assistance programme or counselling services. It is important that you talk to someone as soon as you can, as this will give you the best opportunity of addressing the stressors and prevent significant health conditions arising.

We have previously set out in our mental health chapter some of the adjustments that your employer should consider to help you remain in work, or return to work, if you are suffering from a mental health problem, including stress. The box below describes some of the adjustments that Acas (the Advisory Conciliation and Arbitration Service) suggests that your employer might make. Acas also published new online advice on stress in November 2017, which noted that its helpline dealt with 11,376 calls in 2016 specifically related to stress.[15] The advice noted that Acas's recent research had found that 'emails, in particular, can leave staff feeling overwhelmed if not managed effectively so designing effective systems for prioritizing emails can relieve a lot of work pressures in that area'.

Acas advice on adjustments for staff experiencing mental ill health and stress issues[16]

Adjustments to the work schedule

- Allow more breaks.
- Allow breaks to take place when needed by the team member, rather than on a pre-determined schedule.
- Allow team members to change their working day to start earlier or finish later.

- Allow team members to use paid or unpaid leave for appointments related to their mental health.

- Offer a phased return to work.

- Allow part-time working on a temporary basis (or permanently if it is what the team member wants).

Adjustments to role and responsibilities of a team member

- Review their workload and agree what duties they can do.

- Re-assign duties they may struggle with among the rest of the team.

- Discuss vacant positions in the organization and temporarily transfer the team member to a different role they want to do.

Adjustments to working environment

- Provide partitions, room dividers etc to enhance soundproofing and visual barriers between workspaces.

- Offer a reserved parking space to make it easier for the team member to get to work.

- Offer homeworking for some of the week.

- Increase the size of their 'personal work space'.

- Position the team member as far away as possible from noisy machinery.

- Provide a private space for the team member to use when they need privacy.

Policy changes

- Extend additional paid or unpaid leave during a hospitalization or other absence.

- Allow additional time for the team member to reach performance milestones.

- Allow the team member to make certain personal phone calls during the day.

Ways to provide additional support and assistance

- Assign a mentor or buddy to support and help the team member.
- Arrange a regular one-to-one between the manager and team member to discuss and prioritize tasks.
- Provide a personal computer to enable the team member to work at home when they do not feel able to attend the workplace.
- Offer additional training on the skills the team member's job requires.

The HSE is clear that even where a major influence on the employee's performance and perceptions of work is not work-related, for example caring responsibilities that affect working hours and energy levels, 'it is generally in the employer's interest to support the employee, rather than dismiss the problem as irrelevant to the business'.[17] Again, responses can include adjusting the work or the hours and counselling. Remember, you have the right to request flexible working, which your employer must consider seriously. Although it does not have to agree to flexible working, it can only refuse if there are clear business reasons for so doing.[18]

Further advice

Nearly all trade unions offer excellent advice on stress at work. UNISON, for example, has web pages at www.unison.org.uk/get-help/knowledge/health-and-safety/stress/
Other useful resources include:

Health and Safety Executive: www.hse.gov.uk/stress

Mind: www.mind.org.uk

TUC: www.tuc.org.uk/stress

Stress Management Society: www.stress.org.uk

UK National Work-Stress Network: www.workstress.net

Centre for Stress Management: www.managingstress.com

Anxiety UK: www.anxietyuk.org.uk

Acas: www.acas.org.uk/index.aspx?articleid=6062

National Institute for Health and Care Excellence: www.nice. org.uk/guidance/ph22 (currently being updated)

The British Psychological Society (2017), 'Psychology at work. Improving wellbeing and productivity in the workplace', bit.ly/2JGwGty

Notes

1 www.hse.gov.uk/stress/mental-health.htm

2 HSE (2018) *Health and safety at work. Summary statistics for Great Britain 2017*. bit.ly/2EduV3Y and www.hse.gov.uk/ statistics/causdis/stress

3 www.hse.gov.uk/statistics/causdis/stress/index.htm

4 TUC (2016) *Focus on health and safety. Trade union trends survey. TUC biennial survey of safety reps 2016*, www.tuc.org.uk/ sites/default/files/focusonhealthsafetyreport.pdf

5 HSE (2018) *Summary statistics for Great Britain 2017*

6 HSE (2018) *Summary statistics for Great Britain 2017*

7 www.hse.gov.uk/stress/standards

8 Acas (2014) *Stress at work*

9 www.hse.gov.uk/stress/standards/

10 HSE (2017) *Tackling work-related stress using the management standards approach. A step-by-step workbook*, www.hse.gov.uk/pubns/wbk01.pdf. See also *Work-related stress and how to tackle.* www.hse.gov.uk/stress/what-to-do.htm

11 HSE. *Tackling work-related stress using the management standards approach.* Contains public sector information published by the HSE and licensed under the Open government Licence.

12 Farmer P, Stevenson D (2017) *Thriving at work. The Stevenson/Farmer review of mental health and employers.* bit.ly/2hd3ApX

13 *Stress tools and templates:* www.hse.gov.uk/stress/ standards/downloads.htm

14 HSE. *Tackling work-related stress using the management standards approach*, adapted from appendix 5. www.hse.gov.uk/pubns/wbk01.pdf

15 www.acas.org.uk/index.aspx?articleid=6062

16 www.acas.org.uk/media/pdf/8/5/Common-adjustments-for-staff-experiencing-mental-ill-health.pdf

17 HSE (2017) *Tackling work-related stress using the management standards approach.*

18 *Further advice on flexible working:* www.acas.org.uk/flexibleworking

Chapter 3
Bullying at the workplace and beyond

There is no legal definition of workplace bullying. There is, however, widespread acceptance of what it can entail, including psychological intimidation, persecution, abuse of power, threats and derogatory and denigratory comments. Bullying behaviour also tends to occur persistently and over a period of time (see box). Bullies can be colleagues, contractors, customers, clients or members of the public. Bullying, according to Acas,[1] may be obvious or insidious. The HSE advises, however, that bullies are often more senior than their victims and that they may target groups as well as individuals. A YouGov poll carried out for the TUC in 2015 similarly found that three in four (72%) bullying and harassment incidents were carried out by a manager.

The terms 'harassment' and 'bullying' are often used interchangeably. Harassment, however, has a legal definition under the Equality Act 2010: it is unwanted conduct that has the purpose or effect of violating an individual's dignity or creating an intimidating, hostile, degrading, humiliating or offensive environment for that individual. Crucially, it must be related to a 'protected characteristic', under the Act, ie age, disability, gender reassignment, marriage and civil partnership, pregnancy and maternity, race, religion or belief, sex and sexual orientation.

What is workplace bullying?

Offensive, intimidating, malicious or insulting behaviour, involving an abuse or misuse of power through means intended to undermine, humiliate, denigrate or injure the recipient.

Advisory, Conciliation and Arbitration Service (Acas)

Unlike their playground equivalents workplace bullies and their supporters tend not to use physical abuse. Instead they resort to long term psychological intimidation which can be just as devastating for the person on the receiving end.

National Bullying Helpline[2]

When someone persistently acts in a discriminatory way towards an employee which hurts, criticizes or condemns them.

Mind

A person who deliberately intimidates or persecutes someone they work with.

TUC

There is a wide range of ways in which workplace bullying may manifest at the workplace, although the National Bullying Helpline – which was the first bullying helpline for individuals, including employees – has found that many of its callers do not know whether the behaviour they are experiencing amounts to bullying. Drawing from sources such as the TUC, Acas, anti-bullying advice sites, the HSE and several unions, bullying can manifest as:

- ignoring or excluding a worker, or talking only to a third party to isolate another;
- spreading malicious rumours or gossip;

- humiliating a worker in public;
- giving a worker unachievable or meaningless tasks;
- constantly undervaluing a worker's performance;
- unfairly blaming or victimizing a worker;
- removing areas of responsibility and instead inflicting menial tasks on a worker;
- preventing a worker from progressing, for example by blocking promotion;
- over-bearing supervision;
- racism;
- sexism; and
- unwelcome sexual advances.

The National Bullying Helpline highlights the roles of collusion or exclusion in the workplace in which the behaviour is linked to a group of individuals who are working together.[3] The behaviour may be isolating, intimidating or threatening. 'This behaviour is unacceptable and this group of individuals pose a threat to the organisation as a whole. You need to report this behaviour. An employer is vicariously liable for the unacceptable treatment of one or more persons, provided that treatment is linked,' adds the National Bullying Helpline.

Bullying environments

There are numerous surveys that show that work-related bullying is widespread. The YouGov poll, for example, found that almost three in 10 people (29%) had been bullied at work and that 36% of the victims left their job as a result. The highest prevalence was among women (34% compared with 23% for men) and workers aged between 40 and 59.

The TUC's most recent biennial survey of union safety representatives[4] found that almost half (48%) of respondents listed bullying and harassment as one of their top five concerns in 2016 and that the problem had been 'creeping up' in recent years (41% in 2012). The problem was more pronounced in the public sector than the private sector (53% and 43%) and in workplaces with 200 or more employees than in smaller ones. The sectors with the highest percentages of safety representatives reporting bullying and harassment as a concern were leisure services, central government and education. Dividing employment into 14 broad sectors, bullying and harassment was the:

- most common hazard of concern among representatives in leisure services;
- second most common concern in seven sectors (central government, construction, health services, local government, transport and communications, the voluntary sector and 'other services'); and
- third most common concern in two sectors (education and in banking, insurance and finance).

The TUC argues that the traits of a bully – aggressiveness, sarcasm, anger and maliciousness – flourish in work cultures where:

- the environment is highly competitive or macho;
- the organization is undergoing radical change or cuts;
- jobs are insecure, especially where there is a redundancy threat;
- management styles are tough and hierarchical;
- staff are not involved or consulted about decisions;
- excessive demands are placed on workers; and
- there are no procedures for dealing with bullying.

What can you do?

The effects of bullying can range from few or none, to mild or severe impact on physical and mental health and behaviour to, in the worst cases, suicide. We list in the box some of the effects of bullying and harassment that can beset workers. As with other health conditions in this book, people can have many of these symptoms or traits without suffering from bullying and, as ever, if you are suffering from some of these symptoms, you should always consult your GP to rule out other causes.

Effects of bullying[5]

Physical effects:

- headaches and migraines;
- sweating and shaking;
- feeling sick or vomiting;
- irritable bowels;
- sleep difficulties; and
- loss of appetite.

Mental effects:

- anxiety;
- nervousness;
- panic attacks;
- depression;
- loss of confidence;

- fear of going to work;
- tearfulness; and
- suicidal tendencies.

Behavioural effects:

- irritability;
- becoming withdrawn;
- increased consumption of tobacco, alcohol, etc;
- obsessive dwelling on the bully; and
- seeking justice or revenge (see also box on Post Traumatic Embitterment Disorder).

If you think you may be the victim of bullying, you may be able to deal with the situation informally or you may have to follow a formal procedure. Not all of the suggestions below will be relevant to your individual situation, so pick those that are the best match for you. Some, for example, will be of use only in larger organizations or where trade unions are recognized. You should always, however, gather evidence and talk to people. It is important that you do not resign until you have taken advice.

You should maintain a log of the incidents as they happen. This should include what occurred, who said what, when and where, and who else was present. The log should also include changes to your job, memos and appraisals if relevant to the bullying. Your record should be supported by as much paper and electronic evidence as you can gather. The National Bullying Helpline (NBH)[6] emphasizes that 'it is important to remember that each incident may seem unimportant in isolation but there is a cumulative effect which builds into a much more serious situation'. The experience of the NBH 'is that one of the most distressing parts of being bullied is the feeling that no one seems to care and there is nowhere to go for help.'

The TUC is adamant: 'Don't suffer in silence.'[7] It is vital you speak with one or more of the following:

- Talk to a colleague or a friend who you trust. This can help you think about what to do and also help you cope with any distress you are experiencing.

- If you have a health and safety or union representative, talk to them. If you are not a union member, there may be a staff representative, although they tend not to have as much experience, expertise or support as union representatives, who will have been trained in dealing with such situations and will know the formal procedures and informal ways of dealing with the problem.

- Ask any of your colleagues who have witnessed the bullying behaviour whether they would be prepared to act as witnesses.

- Ask your colleagues whether they are having similar problems. As the TUC noted above, there are particular types of workplaces in which bullying thrives. If you are not the only one suffering from bullying behaviour, a group approach to your employer is likely to be the best way forward.

- Contact a confidential helpline such as Bullying UK,[8] the National Bullying Helpline,[9] the Acas helpline,[10] Citizens Advice, or the Equality and Human Rights Commission (EHRC).[11]

- Talk to someone in your employer's personnel department (there may be a person who deals particularly with equalities).

- Your union might operate a confidential helpline and will almost certainly provide extensive advice on bullying.

- Your employer might offer a helpline through an Employee Assistance Programme (EAP). While this may give you good advice on how to cope and act in the short term, it is not a substitute for your employer addressing the root causes of the bullying.

- Your employer may have 'harassment advisers', who are colleagues who will give you confidential advice.
- Raise the issue with your line manager or supervisor, if appropriate and safe to do so. If the problem involves the line manager, raise it with a more senior manager.

CASE STUDY   Unite bullying and harassment advisors[12]

The joint trade unions working in the forestry industry, and chaired by Unite, decided to act after a staff survey found that 16% of staff (about 500) believed that they had experienced bullying at work in the last two years.

With the support of the employer, unions nominated members as Union bullying and harassment (B&H) advisors. These advisors received formal training on how to handle bullying and harassment and support their members. They now provide a support network right across England, Wales and Scotland. They also meet up to support each other and share information – an essential part of the process.

When it is necessary to take a case to tribunal, advisors support members up to that point then hand over to the full-time union official.

To make it easier for members to report concerns the joint trade unions have circulated practical information leaflets – a *Members' guide to harassment and bullying at work* and a *Quick action guide for union reps.*

The contact details of the union B&H advisors are included on these materials and on the joint trade unions' workplace website; the employer's intranet site has a link direct to this website.

Confronting your bully

Some organizations suggest thinking about talking to the person who is causing you distress. The logic behind this is that an informal chat can prevent a situation escalating and that all the person needs is to be told that the behaviour is distressing. There is also the chance that the person may be unaware or not fully appreciate the effects of their actions. You may believe that it would be pointless to confront informally the person you believe is bullying you but, if you are going to make an approach:

- avoid being alone with the perpetrator at all times and take someone along to the meeting;
- think about what you want the meeting to achieve;
- rehearse with a friend or colleague what you want to say to the bully;
- you or your friend should make a note of the details and the outcomes of the meeting;
- you may prefer to write to the person you feel has been bullying you, either as an alternative to a face-to-face meeting or to set out your feelings in advance of the meeting; and
- you may ask someone else – a colleague, trade union official or counsellor – to act on your behalf and talk to the bully.

Formal procedures

You may need or wish to pursue your bullying allegation formally. If you do so, make sure you are well prepared, have detailed records and evidence, are familiar with your employer's procedures, and are supported by your union representative (or, in the absence of a union, a staff representative or friend). Your employer should:

have a bullying and harassment policy and procedure; promote a culture that does not tolerate bullying and harassment; and be aware of the organizational factors that are associated with bullying and take steps to address them. Check the procedure as it should set out how you can raise your concern and how your employer will respond, as well as stating who is responsible for eliminating bullying. It will also give you information on the emotional support that is available to you and the potential outcomes, including rehabilitation. If your complaint involves changes to your responsibilities, obtain a copy of your job description.

Once you have made a formal complaint, you should expect your employer to investigate quickly and interview you and the alleged bully separately. During your interview, you should again be accompanied by your union representatives or a colleague. Should bullying or harassment be found, action should be taken under your employer's disciplinary procedures. Aside from a warning or even dismissal, additional options can include retraining or relocating the bully.

Post Traumatic Embitterment Disorder

The National Bullying Helpline (NBH) describes Post Traumatic Embitterment Disorder (PTED)[13] as a proposed new disorder that is being diagnosed in the US in relation to workplace harassment and bullying. PTED is modelled after Post Traumatic Stress Disorder (PTSD) but can be clinically separated from it. Sufferers may be less likely to benefit from treatment or medication and instead of being able to deal with the detriment, 'they cannot let go of the feeling of being victimized'.

People with PTED 'can no longer trust anyone around them and the trauma in essence consumes them with a profound "bitterness" making the victim incapable of moving on from the incident. We believe quite a few people are entrapped in their trauma and have been for years.'

The NBH reports 'a lot' of callers to its helpline who 'feel helpless, angry, frustrated or unable to recover from something that happened in the past. We believe this feeling of helplessness and embitterment falls into the PTED category.'

Cyber bullying

Recent years have seen a rising incidence of cyber bullying, which is essentially the use of computers, tablets and smartphones to bully through email, texts, Twitter, Facebook and other social media. Cyber bullying differs from traditional workplace bullying in that it can occur any time, anywhere and anonymously. It can invade your home and other 'safe' and private spaces. It can spread far more rapidly, and to many more people, than in the physical traditional workplace. It can be far harder to control or eliminate once it has occurred and, as Acas notes, can also spill from screen to the workplace and affect interactions with colleagues.[14] A cyber bully may not fit the more common workplace profile of someone in comparative power. In education, for example, it might be a pupil, another teacher or a parent. A 2012 survey by the NASUWT teaching union revealed teachers were facing death threats, accused of crimes, suffering sexist and racist abuse and having their pictures distributed across the net.

If you suffer cyber bullying, take a screen grab of, and print off, any email, text, Facebook entry or other evidence. Do not delete the messages or posts from your phone, tablet or computer. Most of the advice around more traditional workplace bullying still applies, so speak to someone and obtain advice. Compared with more traditional workplace bullying, the evidence may be easier to record and the trail back to the perpetrator easier to identify, although tracing back to the source might not reveal the perpetrator as the account might be hacked, or the phone stolen, etc.

It is also important to ensure that the content is removed. If the perpetrator will not remove the material immediately, you and/or your employer should report it to the site or service host or provider. Further advice can be found in guidance on cyber bullying that the government produced in 2008 with the help of the teaching unions, which also produce their own advice.[15] The Association of Teachers and Lecturers (now part of the National Education Union), for example, produced a 2014 cyber bullying factsheet[16] that emphasizes the need to check that the website or social media platform has actually made the requested amendments or removals and that, if it does not cooperate, the victim's senior manager should contact the internet service provider, which can block access to pages and even close down a website. You should also ensure that a website 'uncaches' pages because, even after they have been removed, they will be stored (cached) and detectable by search engines. Facebook has advice on bullying, although this is not specifically concerned with employment other than in education.[17] It does, however, have advice on reporting abuse.[18] Acas also has a page dedicated to cyber bullying.[19]

Legal redress

There are various legal routes open to you for redress and/or compensation. Before you embark on any such course, take advice from your union representative, a Citizens Advice (CAB) or a lawyer:

- Discrimination under the Equality Act 2010, if the harassment or bullying relates to a protected characteristic (see case study on page 191). You can get advice and help from the Equality Advisory and Support Service, including on how to apply to an employment tribunal.[20]

- If you have suffered a mental health condition (for example anxiety) or physical injury as a result of your employer's breach of its duty of care to you or its statutory duties, you may be able to sue for compensation in the civil courts.

- If you have left your job because conditions have become so bad that you cannot continue, you might be able to claim for constructive dismissal, again at an employment tribunal. This, according to the TUC's website should only be a last resort and is 'a high-risk strategy with many potential pitfalls'. You would need to act within three months of your last day of work and be able to show that your employer's failure to take action involved a serious or fundamental breach of contract, for example by failing to investigate your allegation properly, or by failing to provide a safe place of work. You would also need to have been employed for two years. Remember, constructive dismissal claims are very hard to win. Your colleagues might not be willing to give evidence and even if the tribunal finds your employer's behaviour was unacceptable, it may still decide that its behaviour following the incident – for example, in apologizing – 'repaired' the fundamental breach.

Notes

1 Acas (2014) *Bullying and harassment at work. A guide for employees*. www.acas.org.uk/media/pdf/r/l/Bullying-and-harassment-at-work-a-guide-for-employees.pdf

2 nationalbullyinghelpline.co.uk/employees.html

3 nationalbullyinghelpline.co.uk/employees.html

4 TUC (2016) *Focus on health and safety. Trade union trends survey. TUC biennial survey of safety reps 2016,* www.tuc.org.uk/ sites/default/files/focusonhealthsafetyreport.pdf

5 These are drawn mainly from the TUC's advice and supplemented from other sources.

6 nationalbullyinghelpline.co.uk/employees.html

7 TUC, *Bullying, violence and harassment,* www.tuc.org.uk/ workplace-guidance/bullying-violence-and-harassment

8 www.bullying.co.uk, tel: 0808 800 2222

9 National Bullying Helpline, tel: 0845 2255 787

10 Acas helpline, tel: 0300 123 11 00

11 www.equalityhumanrights.com

12 Reproduced from Unite, *Health and safety guide,* www.unitetheunion.org/uploaded/documents/Bullying,%20 harassment%20%26%20violence%20in%20the%20 workplace%20(Unite%20guide)11-5110.pdf

13 nationalbullyinghelpline.co.uk/employees.html

14 Acas, *Cyber bullying,* www.acas.org.uk/index.aspx? articleid=3379

15 Department for Children, Schools and Families (2008), *Cyber bullying: Supporting staff,* www.digizen.org/downloads/ cyberbullying_teachers.pdf

16 ATL (2014) *Cyber bullying,* www.atl.org.uk/advice-and-resources/ publications/cyberbullying

17 *Put a stop to bullying,* www.facebook.com/safety/bullying

18 www.facebook.com/help/1753719584844061?helpref=h
c_global_nav

19 www.acas.org.uk/index.aspx?articleid=3379

20 Equality Advisory and Support Service, tel: 0808 800 0082

Chapter 4
Suicide

Almost 6,000 people die by suicide in the UK each year but, until recently, it has been ignored as a workplace issue.[1] Now, many organizations, business leaders and trade unions are speaking out. Their message is that suicide is not inevitable; it is preventable. By creating more open, supportive working environments we can all help to reduce the risk of death by suicide.

Suicide is a workplace issue

Despite being neglected as a workplace issue (even RIDDOR, the regulations that govern reporting accidents at work, specifically exclude suicide), there are important reasons why suicide should be seen in the context of work.

First, poor workplaces are bad for our mental health. Precarious work, impossible targets, bullying and harassment can be major sources of stress (see chapters 2 and 3). And poor employers who ignore these stressors are much less likely to provide the effective leadership, training and support that can help prevent suicide.

Second, preventing suicide requires action by employers and colleagues as well as friends, family and healthcare professionals. People with jobs spend around one-third of their life at work, so workplaces provide important opportunities to reach people who are in distress and may be thinking of suicide.

Third, good working conditions can actively help prevent suicide. Employers need to create a supportive working environment, one where people feel able to talk about difficult issues, where managers are trained to spot early warning signs and where everyone knows where to get the help they need.

Some background

Today, we are beginning to talk more openly about suicide both in and outside the workplace. That's important because one in five of us will have suicidal thoughts sometime in our lives. The UK government now has a national strategy that aims to reduce suicide by 10% by 2020–21. Suicide is preventable, but preventing suicide is about more than governments and targets: to prevent suicides at work, we all can and need to do more.

In 2016 (the latest year that data are available) 5,965 people died by suicide in the UK – that's more than 16 people each day. Every suicide is a tragedy for the individual, their family and their work colleagues. But behind the headline figures, there are some big differences in suicide rates among different parts of the population.[2]

Suicide is the main cause of death for men under the age of 50. Although women are less at risk, the rate of female suicide is the highest it has been for more than a decade. The risk of suicide is higher among the lesbian, gay, bisexual and transgender community, and for people who are unemployed.

When the UK's Office for National Statistics analysed suicide rates by occupation, they found some striking differences. For men, those most at risk are construction workers, while among women, nurses, primary school teaches and those in media, culture and sport have above-average suicide rates. Among both men and women, care workers have a risk of suicide double the national average.[3]

Inequality impacts suicide rates, and people who live in deprived areas are more at risk. Research commissioned by Samaritans concluded that job insecurity, zero-hours contracts and economic recession can all increase the risk of suicide.[4]

CASE STUDY   Mates in Construction

In Australia, construction workers are six times more likely to die from suicide than from an accident at work.[5] Mates in Construction (MIC) was set up in 2008 to reduce this death toll. MIC commissioned research that showed that construction workers found it hard to discuss their feelings with colleagues at work, either because the nature of the work made social support more difficult or because they felt that admitting to problems was 'not manly'.

MIC is an integrated training and support programme aimed at raising awareness about suicide at work, making it easy to access help, and ensuring that help is practical, professional and appropriate. By 2016, MIC had provided training and support to 100,000 construction workers.

matesinconstruction.org.au

The causes

Suicide is complex and there is no single reason why people take their own lives. Many factors – psychological and social as well as economic and cultural – interact to increase a person's risk of suicide. Suicide usually occurs gradually, progressing from suicidal thoughts, to planning, attempting suicide and finally dying by suicide.[6]

In explaining death by suicide, the focus has tended to be on a person's mental health. While mental illness is an underlying factor in most suicides, the picture is much more complex and is not fully understood.

Men from disadvantaged backgrounds in their 30s, 40s and 50s are at highest risk of suicide, and research by Samaritans found that many factors are involved. These include certain personality traits, ideas about masculinity, challenges of mid-life, relationship breakdown, socioeconomic factors, drug and alcohol misuse, and attitudes to support services.[7]

And although attitudes to mental health are changing, mental health at work is still stigmatized and this is a barrier to people getting the help and support they need (see chapter 1).

Creating healthier workplaces

There are many simple, practical things we can all do at work to help prevent suicide. Some – such as having the right policies and procedures in place, tackling workplace stress, preventing bullying and harassment, and providing psychological support services – are your employer's responsibility. Other things, such as talking and being aware of the danger signs, everyone can do. However, remember that while you can help prevent suicide, you are not responsible for other people's actions.

According to Business in the Community's suicide prevention toolkit,[8] elements of a workplace suicide prevention plan might include:

- a supportive workplace culture that fosters open communication;

- mental health and suicide prevention training for staff, especially line managers;

- clear policies on mental health and other factors that can increase the risk of suicide;

- clear signposting to support services like Samaritans;

- a plan for responding to a suicide attempt or death.

Talking more about suicide is one of the most important things you can do. According to Poppy Jarvis of Mental Health First Aid England: 'The biggest myth we need to bust is that talking about suicide increases the risk of someone taking their own life, when in reality talking is the most powerful first step towards safety, yet the hardest thing to do when we are distressed.'[9]

Although talking is the vital first step to getting help, discussing suicide is difficult. It helps if your workplace culture is one of openness and respect. This makes it more likely that people will feel able to talk about feeling overwhelmed or having suicidal thoughts. Helping people talk about these feelings, either with a manager or work colleague, is an opportunity to help people get support.

Talking more openly can also help reduce the stigma that still surrounds suicide, and so can good leadership. Paul Polman, CEO of Unilever, wants more business leaders to ensure that they have action plans in place that address mental ill health and wellbeing at work. 'We must give people the confidence to step forward to ask for help, and equip managers with the skills needed to respond effectively. Nobody should be more than one call, one click or one chat away from help,' he says.

CASE STUDY   University of Cambridge Clinical School Wellbeing Programme

The University of Cambridge Clinical School has run a wellbeing programme since 2015. As well as physical health (30-minute health checks, nutrition talks, walking challenges and a dedicated wellbeing website and newsletter), the programme includes a range of mental health elements, including lunchtime briefings for staff, Mental Health First Aid training for managers, an annual Mental Health Awareness Week, and wellbeing recovery plans to support staff with bipolar disorder and other conditions.

The Clinical School has also signed the STOP Suicide organizational pledge (a Cambridgeshire-wide initiative for individuals and organizations), trained 10 Mental Health First Aiders and provided mental health crisis and suicide prevention training for staff and first aiders.

Feedback has been overwhelmingly positive, and a survey showed that 71 per cent of staff knew where to find support services for wellbeing and mental ill health.

According to HR Business Manager Caroline Newman, who set up the programme:

> We need to dispel myths about mental health and illness. We spend so much time at work that our wellbeing at work is intimately linked with our home life. We're trying to cascade the message that whether you've got anxiety, or depression, or a more severe condition, it's OK. We know people can function well but, at certain points, they may need more support.

University of Cambridge Clinical School Wellbeing Programme
www.medschl.cam.ac.uk/human-resources/staff-wellbeing

While we're on the subject of talking, it's worth remembering that some people find it much harder to talk than others. It seems like a stereotype, but men can find it harder to talk about how they are feeling than women. Several grass-roots initiatives have sprung up to meet this need, including Mates in Construction (see case study) and the Men's Sheds movement, both of which began in Australia but are spreading worldwide. Men's Sheds arrived in the UK in 2013; today, there are more than 400 sheds across the UK where 10,000 'shedders' connect, converse and create, and in 2017 the UK construction industry set up Mates in Mind to raise awareness of mental health.

Awareness is vital. Understanding suicidal thoughts and behaviour means you're more likely to be able to intervene before it's too late. As well as creating a supportive work culture, managers need training so that they can spot early warning signs and support people to get the help they need. The idea of mental health first aid (MHFA) training began in Australia in 2000 and since then more than two million people have been trained in MHFA skills worldwide. MHFA

England was set up in 2007 and provides training for individuals and organizations. You can find out more about these courses at the MHFA England website.[10]

CASE STUDY   Cornwall Council

Cornwall Council's Health Promotion Service[11] provides three training courses to give people who live or work in Cornwall and the Isles of Scilly the necessary tools to save a life from suicide. 'People who die from suicide are not always in contact with health services, yet they often continue to go to work even as their ability to cope deteriorates,' the Council says. More than two-thirds of people are in employment, so the workplace offers a practical opportunity to reach people who need support and to reduce stigma around mental health.

ASIST (which stands for Applied Suicide Intervention Skills Training) is two-day workshop that teaches people how to recognize when someone may have thoughts of suicide, and work with them to create a plan that will support their immediate safety. Since it was developed in 1983 by a US suicide intervention company called LivingWorks, more than one million people have completed the ASIST workshop.

SuicideTALK is a 90-minute presentation aimed at building awareness of suicide prevention. It deals openly with the stigma that surrounds suicide, and by asking participants 'should we talk about suicide?' it unpacks personal and social beliefs about suicide.

SafeTALK is a half-day training course aimed at making a difference in the workplace. It complements the ASIST workshop, and equips people with the tools to give immediate support to someone having thoughts of suicide and to signpost sources of specialist help.

Knowing who to contact if someone is in distress is also important. In larger businesses this may be occupational health departments and EAPs (see chapter 12), a GP or confidential helpline such as Samaritans.

While we know that suicide is a gradual process, the actual decision to do so can be impulsive. Research shows that people are less likely to die by suicide if they do not have the means to do so. This is called 'means restriction' and should be part of workplace risk assessments.

Trade union representatives can also play a role, and TUC guidance highlights several things that workplace reps can do. These include making sure your employer views suicide as a workplace issue and provides access to help and support, and jointly reviewing your employer's policies on stress, bullying and harassment, mental health and employee assistance.[12]

Suicide in the workplace is very uncommon, but it's good practice for employers to have plans in place to provide the right care for those affected. These interventions are sometimes called 'postvention' and Business in the Community has produced a free postvention toolkit for employers.[13]

Warning signs

Not everyone who is thinking about suicide will display warning signs, but there can be behavioural signals. You may notice differences such as a decline in work output or quality; they may start being late or missing work or find it hard to concentrate and complete work. They may become more withdrawn or isolated, and their behaviour may change. They may, for example, become more anxious, agitated or angry, have mood swings or start behaving recklessly. Or their eating patterns may change, they might increase the amount of alcohol or drugs they use, or you might notice signs that someone is self-harming.

How to respond to warning signs

If you are worried about someone at work, you can take the following steps, depending on what feels most comfortable to you.

1 Talk with your line manager, HR, occupational health department or EAP, or call Samaritans for emotional support.

2 Reach out to the person:

   - Ask how he or she is doing.

   - Listen without judging.

   - Mention changes you have noticed in the person's behaviour and say that you are concerned about their wellbeing.

   - Suggest that he or she talk with someone in the EAP, HR, occupational health department, or another health professional, such as their GP. Signpost to helplines like Samaritans and CALM.

   - Continue to provide support; make it clear that you will always be willing to listen.

   - Always follow up with other people where possible to ensure that action has been taken.

What to do in a crisis

Take action if you encounter someone who is at immediate risk. This is very similar to what you would do if you came across a colleague who had had a physical accident or health issue like chest pain.

Take the following steps right away:

1 If the danger for self-harm seems imminent, make sure the person is not left alone and call 999.

2 Stay with the person (or make sure the person is in a private, secure place with another caring person) until professional help arrives.

3 Encourage the person to talk but do not promise to keep the conversation confidential.

4 Ask the person if there is anyone they would like to call such as Samaritans, their GP or mental health professional. If they agree, give them space (and perhaps if they need it, help them call Samaritans) so that they have someone to talk to immediately.

5 Contact the HR Department, OHS or EAP, depending on company policy, to let them know what is happening.

6 Once the person is under the care of a professional, agree if they would like you to stay with them or not. Follow up with HR, OHS or EAP as appropriate.

7 Get support for yourself. Don't underestimate the impact this can have on yourself once the immediate risk has passed.

It is better to over-react than to later ask yourself whether you could have done more. But whatever happens, do not feel guilty. You can play an important role in preventing suicide but you are not responsible for other people's actions.

Where to get help

Samaritans' free 24-hour helpline, tel: 116 123, www.samaritans.org

UK Men's Sheds Association menssheds.org.uk

Mates in Mind www.matesinmind.org

CALM www.thecalmzone.net

Notes

1 ONS (2017) *Suicides in the UK: 2016 registrations.*
www.ons.gov.uk/peoplepopulationandcommunity/
birthsdeathsandmarriages/deaths/bulletins/suicidesintheunitedking
dom/2016registrations

2 Ibid.

3 ONS (2017) *Suicide by occupation, England: 2011 to 2015.*
www.ons.gov.uk/peoplepopulationandcommunity/
birthsdeathsandmarriages/deaths/articles/suicidebyoccupation/
england2011to2015

4 Samaritans (2017) *Suicide statistics report 2017.* www.samaritans.
org/about-us/our-research/facts-and-figures-about-suicide

5 Milner A et al. (2017) *Male suicide among construction workers in
Australia: a qualitative analysis of the major stressors precipitating
death*, BMC Public Health, **17**, p. 584. https://bmcpublichealth.
biomedcentral.com/articles/10.1186/s12889-017-4500-8

6 Samaritans (2017) *Dying from inequality.* www.samaritans.org/
sites/default/files/kcfinder/files/Samaritans%20Dying%20from%20
inequality%20report%20-%20summary.pdf

7 Samaritans (2012) *Men and suicide.* www.samaritans.org/sites/
default/files/kcfinder/files/Samaritans_Men_and_Suicide_Report_
web.pdf

8 Business in the Community (2017) *Reducing the risk of suicide:
a toolkit for employers.* https://wellbeing.bitc.org.uk/sites/
default/files/business_in_the_community_suicide_prevention_
toolkit_0.pdf

9 MHFA (2017) *Suicide Prevention Toolkit published to support
employers.* https://mhfaengland.org/mhfa-centre/news/
2017-03-17-suicide-prevention-toolkit-published-to-support-em

10 https://mhfaengland.org

11 Cornwall Council Health Promotion Service:
www.healthpromcornwall.org

12 TUC (2018) *Work and suicide: A TUC guide to prevention for
trade union activists.* www.tuc.org.uk/sites/default/files/work-and-
suicide.pdf

13 BITC (2017) *Reducing the risk of suicide*

Chapter 5
Occupational cancers

When cancers are caused by people's work, they are called occupational cancers. Occupational cancers can be caused by many things, and affect many workers, but despite this they have often been overlooked. As a result, occupational cancer is sometimes referred to as a 'forgotten epidemic'. This chapter explains how work can cause cancer and what your employer must do to protect you.

Cancer: some definitions

What we commonly refer to as one disease – cancer – is actually dozens of different diseases, caused by various things and affecting different parts of the body. In fact, there are more than 200 different types of cancer.

Cancers can be categorized in several different ways. They are often grouped according to where in the body they start, such as the breast or the prostate. They are also grouped according to the type of cell that they begin in. Looked at this way, there are five main groups of cancer, dependent on what part of the body they affect: the skin or tissues around internal organs (carcinomas), connective tissues like bone or muscle (sarcomas), blood-forming tissue like bone marrow (leukaemias), the immune system (lymphoma and myeloma) and the brain and spinal cord (central nervous system cancers).[1]

Cancer is a genetic disease. This means that it's caused by changes, or mutations, in the genes that control how our cells function. Many things can cause mutations, from tobacco smoking and ionizing radiation to ultraviolet rays in sunlight and environmental chemicals. All these things can increase our risk of developing cancer and it's thought that they account for around 90% of cancers, while only 10% come from faulty genes inherited from our parents.[2]

Cancer is also a multifactorial disease. This means that rather than having one single cause, most cancers result from the combined effects of several different things. When these result from workplace exposures – which are discussed below – we call these work-related or occupational cancers.

Occupational cancer: the scale of the problem

Around the world, it's estimated that 666,000 people every year die due to work-related cancers. Asbestos is the biggest killer, but there are many others, from diesel fumes and silica dust to solar radiation. In the UK, the Health and Safety Executive (HSE) estimates that around 13,500 of the new cases of cancer that occur every year are the result of people's work, and that 8,000 people die each year due to occupational cancers. And in the European Union as a whole, some 102,000 deaths a year are due to occupational cancer, making it the leading cause of death across the EU.[3]

When you compare this death toll to the number of workplace deaths due to accidents, the scale of the problem becomes clear. In 2017/18, 144 workers were killed in workplace accidents in Great Britain. Around 40 times as many are dying as a result of occupational cancers.[4]

Even this number could be an underestimate. The reason why we do not have accurate data on the scale of the problem is because while fatal accidents are accurately recorded, the same is not true for occupational cancer. Cancers take many years to develop, a time lag which doctors call a latency period. For leukaemia and other blood cancers, this latency period can be 20 years, but for other forms of cancer it can be up to 50 years. That means that if you are diagnosed with cancer today, it could have been caused by occupational exposures some time in the past five decades. Because most of us change jobs and employers several times during our lives, it's very difficult to work out how many cancers are caused by work.

Another reason for the lack of accurate figures on workplace cancers is that it is almost always impossible to state accurately that an individual cancer is caused by exposure to a specific substance. Even if the link can be shown, such as that between skin cancer and excessive sun exposure, proving that the cause is occupational is difficult as people are exposed to sun on holiday as well as at work.

As a result, the TUC argues that the true level is likely to be well over 20,000 cases a year with 15,000–18,000 deaths. However, rather than debating about whether it's 8,000 or 18,000, we should be focusing on the fact that all occupational cancers are avoidable.[5]

Asbestos: killer dust

Asbestos is the world's biggest ever industrial killer, and the single greatest cause of work-related deaths in the UK. Asbestos-related diseases kill around 5,500 people a year in Great Britain. The vast majority of these deaths are due to occupational cancer, including 2,542 mesothelioma deaths, 2,500 due to asbestos-related lung cancer, and around 90 deaths from laryngeal, ovarian and stomach cancer caused by asbestos.

Although asbestos is banned in 55 countries around the world, including the UK, the problem has not gone away. In Britain, deaths from mesothelioma and other asbestos-related diseases will not start to decline until 2020 because of past working conditions. And although more than 1.3 million tradespeople are at risk from asbestos, there is a clear lack of awareness about it. According to an HSE survey of 500 tradespeople in 2014, only 30% could identify all the correct measures for working safely with asbestos.

Asbestos – a group of naturally occurring fibrous minerals which comes in different forms, often referred to as white, blue and brown asbestos – has been killing people for many years and will continue to do so.

Used for thousands of years, asbestos began to be mined for large-scale industrial use from the 1880s. Because of its physical properties – it is strong, hard-wearing, flexible but above all insulating and fire-resistant – it was used in thousands of products across many industries, from building insulation to the car industry. By 1975, around five million tons of asbestos were mined around the world, with the USA, Canada, Australia and South Africa among the major producers.

Although construction workers are most at risk, other groups are also exposed to asbestos at work. Since 1980, at least 319 teachers have died from mesothelioma, for example.

After many years of campaigning, brown and blue asbestos was banned in the UK in 1985 and white asbestos was finally banned in 1999. Although it is now illegal to use asbestos in construction or refurbishment of any premises, thousands of tonnes of it remain in all buildings built before 2000. There are a number of resources available that give more information on managing asbestos in buildings, including:

www.hse.gov.uk/toolbox/harmful/asbestos.htm

www.mesothelioma.uk.com

HSE: Asbestos-related diseases. www.hse.gov.uk/statistics/
    causdis/asbestosis/asbestos-related-disease.pdf

http://www.hse.gov.uk/construction/healthrisks/cancer-and-
    construction/asbestos.htm

NUT: www.teachers.org.uk/edufacts/asbestos

TUC: Asbestos: Time to get rid of it. Available at www.tuc.org.uk/
    research-analysis/reports/asbestos-%E2%80%93-time-get-rid-it

Hazards: Asbestos figures. Available at www.hazards.org/
    asbestos/asbestosfigures.htm

What causes occupational cancers?

Although the numbers are challenging to pin down, we know plenty about the kind of workplace exposures that can cause cancer. Things that cause cancer are called carcinogens, and there are three different types of occupational carcinogen. We often associate cancer with chemicals. Those that cause cancer – and which can be commonly encountered at work – include naturally occurring substances like asbestos, as well as man-made chemicals such as vinyl chloride or the by-products of particular manufacturing processes. But chemicals are only part of the picture.

As well as chemical carcinogens, there are physical carcinogens such as ionizing and ultraviolet radiation, and biological carcinogens. Exposing your skin to too much UV radiation is the main cause of skin cancer. Viruses can cause cancer directly or indirectly, for example by causing chronic inflammation (such as hepatitis B) or suppressing the body's immune system (HIV). Certain working patterns also increase the risk of cancer; long-term night shift work, for example, is associated with increased risk of breast, skin and digestive system cancers in women.

Much of what we know about occupational carcinogens comes from studying the number and kinds of cancers in different groups of workers. From this, we know that many workplace exposures – from wood dust and radon to arsenic and metalworking fluids – can cause cancer. We can also make judgements based on what we know from laboratory experiments on cells in test tubes and in animal studies.

IARC – the International Agency for Research on Cancer[6] – is part of the World Health Organization. IARC was set up in 1965 and today has members from 25 countries around the world. Its job is to promote international collaboration in cancer research and to examine all the scientific evidence to decide whether or not something causes cancer. IARC publishes these evaluations in a series of monographs and, depending on the weight of evidence, divides carcinogens into several categories.

If there is enough evidence that something causes cancer in humans, it's described as a Group 1 carcinogen. There are currently 120 agents in this group, and they include specific chemicals such as benzene and formaldehyde, groups of metallic compounds such as nickel and cadmium, industrial processes such as rubber manufacturing, occupational groups such as painters, and environmental exposures from alcohol consumption to tobacco smoking.

Where the evidence is less strong, substances are classified as Group 2A (probably carcinogenic to humans) or Group 2B (possibly carcinogenic to humans). Where there is too little information available, it's put into Group 3 (not classifiable as to its carcinogenicity to humans). In total, according to IARC, there are more than 50 occupational carcinogens that fall into groups 1 and 2A, with another 100 in Group 2B.[7]

Who is most at risk?

Given the kind of exposures involved, large differences exist in the risk of occupational cancer in different jobs. Research by the HSE shows that past occupational exposure to asbestos is the leading cause of workplace cancer, accounting for some 4,000 deaths in 2005. Half of these were due to mesothelioma and the other half to lung cancer, which means asbestos caused one in every two occupational deaths in 2005. Since then, asbestos-related cancer deaths have increased by about to around 5,000 per year and the HSE thinks that mesothelioma deaths will not start to decline until 2020.[8]

As well as asbestos, other major occupational carcinogens include silica, diesel engine exhausts and mineral oils (in terms of their contribution to cancer deaths), and shift-working, mineral oils and solar radiation (in terms of their contribution to new cases of cancer).[9]

Because of exposure to asbestos and silica, the construction industry has the largest burden of occupational cancer in Britain.

Research by the HSE shows that around 3,500 construction workers die each year due to occupational cancer, with another 5,500 being diagnosed with occupational cancer. This means that more than 40% of all occupational cancer deaths and new cases of occupational cancer occur in construction – around 100 times more than the number of construction workers killed in accidents at work.[10]

Carcinogens, hazardous substances and the law

COSHH – or the Control of Substances Hazardous to Health Regulations 2002 – is the law that requires employers to control substances that are hazardous to health. Your employer should prevent or reduce exposure to hazardous substances by:

- finding out what the health hazards are;
- deciding how to prevent harm to health (risk assessment);
- providing control measures to reduce harm to health;
- making sure control measures are used;
- keeping all control measures in good working order;
- providing information, instruction and training for employees and others;
- providing monitoring and health surveillance in appropriate cases;
- planning for emergencies.

In 2018, the European Commission introduced new legislation on workplace carcinogens and outlined new plans to strictly limit exposure to five carcinogens including cadmium, beryllium and formaldehyde.

HSE www.hse.gov.uk/coshh/basics.htm

European Commission: http://europa.eu/rapid/press-release_IP-18-2662_en.htm

Preventing occupational cancers

Your employer has a legal duty, as far as is reasonably practicable, to ensure your health at work. As well as this general duty under the Health and Safety at Work Act 1974, the Management of Health and Safety at Work Regulations 1999 also require employers to conduct a suitable assessment of risks to the health of the workforce. That includes any risk from any hazard that may cause cancer (see chapter 19).

As well as these general duties, the principal piece of legislation that covers hazardous substances at work is the Control of Substances Hazardous to Health Regulations 2002 or COSHH for short (see box). Special legislation, the Control of Asbestos Regulations 2012, covers asbestos.

Carcinogens, like other hazardous substances, can find their way into your body via several routes – through the skin, by being breathed in or by being swallowed. Because many occupational diseases like cancer take a long time to develop, preventing workplace exposure is key to preventing them.

Controlling exposure to hazardous substances at work is done through a system of exposure limits. In the UK these are called workplace exposure limits (WELs). These are legal limits on the amount of a particular substance that can be present in workplace air. They are set by one of the European Commission's scientific committees, which examine the scientific information on the health effects of hundreds of hazardous substances, and are published by the HSE in a list called EH40.[11]

However, cancer is such a serious disease that the law treats carcinogens differently to other hazardous substances at work. This is based on the premise that there is no safe level of exposure to a carcinogen, so the law says that for substances that cause cancer (or asthma), your employer must reduce levels 'as far as is reasonably practicable'.

The law also tells employers how they should control exposure to carcinogens at work. Known as a hierarchy of controls, this means there are certain things an employer must do first. First and foremost, they should eliminate the hazard by substituting the carcinogen for a safer substance. If this is not possible, then they should use engineering controls to enclose the process or local exhaust ventilation to remove a carcinogen from the air. Personal protective equipment (PPE) is a last resort. This is because PPE is often unreliable, only partially effective, or not used properly. Unfortunately, according to the TUC, many employers go straight to this option rather than removing or reducing exposure to a carcinogen by other means.

Because there is no safe limit for carcinogens, trade unions have always argued that there should be no workplace exposure to anything that causes cancer. 'Where possible this will mean removing carcinogens from the workplace completely,' says the TUC. 'In some cases that is not practical, but in these cases the worker should be fully protected from exposure.' These cases include radiographers (who work with ionizing radiation), quarry workers (who work with silica) and bus mechanics (who work with diesel exhaust).[12]

As well as controlling exposure, employers have a legal duty to carry out appropriate health surveillance of workers exposed to certain substances. These are listed in the COSHH Regulations but any worker exposed to any possible carcinogen should be regularly monitored to ensure there are no adverse health effects arising from the exposure.

As well as the law, there are several campaigns that you or your trade union could encourage your employer to join. Launched in 2014 by IOSH to raise awareness of occupational cancer, the No Time to Lose campaign provides employers with free resources on asbestos, silica dust, solar radiation and diesel exhaust emissions and asks employers to pledge to promote positive change at work. More than 100 organizations have done so, using a six-step plan to note what they're doing to manage exposures to carcinogens at work.[13]

For some types of occupational cancer you are entitled to benefits under the Industrial Injuries Scheme. Most occupational cancer cases compensated by the scheme are related to asbestos exposure, but as well as mesothelioma and lung cancer due to asbestos, several other occupational cancers are covered. These include skin cancers due to workplace exposure to arsenic, soot or mineral oils, bladder cancer due to certain workplace chemicals and liver cancer due to chemicals used in PVC manufacture. You can find a full list of these so-called prescribed diseases, and how to claim, on the internet.[14]

If you are concerned about workplace carcinogens, you should speak to your trade union rep, your occupational health department or report it to the HSE.

Notes

1 CRUK. *What is cancer?* www.cancerresearchuk.org/about-cancer/ what-is-cancer

2 National Cancer Institute. *The genetics of cancer.* www.cancer.gov/ about-cancer/causes-prevention/genetics

3 ETUI (2017) *Occupational cancers.* www.etui.org/Topics/Health-Safety-working-conditions/Occupational-cancers

4 See HSE (2018), Workplace fatal injuries in Great Britain 2018. www.hse.gov.uk/statistics/pdf/fatalinjuries.pdf. www.hse.gov.uk/ statistics/pdf/fatalinjuries.pdf and HSE (2017), *Occupational Cancer in Great Britain.* www.hse.gov.uk/statistics/causdis/cancer/ cancer.pdf?pdf=cancer

5 TUC (2012) *Occupational cancer: a workplace guide.* www.tuc. org.uk/sites/default/files/occupationalcancer.pdf

6 IARC: www.iarc.fr

7 IARC (2006) IARC monographs on the evaluation of carcinogenic risks to humans. http://monographs.iarc.fr/ENG/Preamble/ CurrentPreamble.pdf

8 HSE (2017) Asbestos-related diseases. www.hse.gov.uk/statistics/causdis/asbestosis/asbestos-related-disease.pdf

9 HSE (2017) Occupational Cancer in Great Britain. www.hse.gov.uk/statistics/causdis/cancer/cancer.pdf?pdf=cancer.

10 HSE (2017) Occupational Cancer in Great Britain. www.hse.gov.uk/statistics/causdis/cancer/cancer.pdf?pdf=cancer and the accidents part to Health and Safety Executive (2017) Fatal injuries arising from accidents at work in Great Britain 2017. www.hse.gov.uk/statistics/pdf/fatalinjuries.pdf

11 HSE (2011) EH40/2005 Workplace exposure limits. www.hse.gov.uk/pubns/books/eh40.htm

12 TUC (2012) *Occupational cancer*. See also International Metalworkers' Federation (2007), *Occupational cancer/zero cancer: A union guide to prevention*. www.hazards.org/cancer/preventionkit/docs/ZeroCancer_en.pdf

13 IOSH. *No time to lose*. Available at www.notimetolose.org.uk

14 DWP (2017) *Industrial Injuries Disablement Benefits: technical guidance*. www.gov.uk/government/publications/industrial-injuries-disablement-benefits-technical-guidance/industrial-injuries-disablement-benefits-technical-guidance#prescribed-diseases

Chapter 6
Musculoskeletal disorders

Musculoskeletal disorders (or musculoskeletal conditions, as they are increasingly referred to) is the term used to describe a variety of painful conditions that affect the muscles and joints – for example, bad backs and repetitive strain injury (RSI). And they affect millions of people; in England alone, it's estimated that 17% of people of all ages have back pain. Poorly designed and repetitive work is an important cause of musculoskeletal disorders (MSDs), which is why making workplaces healthier can help to prevent the pain and time off work that they cause.

Millions like us

Work-related MSDs are the most common cause of occupational ill health in Great Britain. In 2016/17, more than half a million workers suffered from MSDs caused – or made worse – by their work. Around 194,000 of these had bad backs, 229,000 had hand, arm or neck problems and another 84,000 had lower limb problems.[1]

Many people have to take time off work as a result. Looking at MSDs as a whole, they accounted for some 30.8 million days off work in 2016 – that's more than two in 10 of all sick days and second only to minor illnesses like coughs and colds.[2] When it comes to work-related ill health, their impact is even greater. In 2016/17, around 8.9 million working days were lost due to work-related MSDs – that's four out of every 10 working days lost because of work-related ill health.[3]

Between 1990 and 2016, lower back pain and neck pain were the leading causes of disability in England.[4] Because of the huge scale of the problem, the Health and Safety Executive has made MSDs (along with occupational stress and cancers – see chapters 2 and 5) one of its three key priorities.

In Europe as a whole, it's estimated that MSDs cost employers, workers and health services €163 billion a year, and the European Trade Union Confederation is calling on the European Commission to do more to tackle what it calls an 'epidemic of back, shoulder, neck, elbow, hand and knee pain costing workers severe loss of quality of life and millions of days off work'.[5] But, it's important to remember that occasional aches and pains are part of everyday life. If you rest, your body will be able to recover on its own.

What are musculoskeletal disorders?

The term 'musculoskeletal disorder' is an umbrella term used to describe the huge range of often painful disorders that affect our bones, soft tissues, and their nerves. Because it's such a broad term, it's often subdivided in various ways.

It can be categorized by the area of the body that's affected: upper limb disorders (ULDs) are things that affect our necks, arms and hands; lower limb disorders (LLDs) refer to things that affect our hips, legs, knees, ankles and feet; and others, of course, affect our backs.

Examples of ULDs are specific medical conditions such as carpal tunnel syndrome and frozen shoulder, and other painful conditions like RSI. LLDs include conditions such as osteoarthritis in the knees or hips

These conditions can also be subdivided in a way that reflects their cause. Some MSDs may be caused by things we do outside work, such as our hobbies and the sports we play, and other aspects of our lifestyle, such as how active we are and whether we're a healthy weight. Others are caused (or made worse) by work, and these are described as work-related MSDs.

Lastly, MSDs can be divided more medically according to whether they involve inflammation (such as rheumatoid arthritis), pain (for example osteoarthritis or back pain), or osteoporosis or fractures.[6]

Whatever their cause or location, the kind of symptoms associated with MSDs are pain, swelling, tingling, numbness, weakness and stiffness. Although most people assume that the symptoms of MSDs are physical, it's also worth knowing that MSDs are often associated with depression. When researchers studied people who were off work due to MSDs, they found that by 12 months after the injury, almost 30% of people were being treated for depression.[7]

This study highlights that when you are off work for a significant period of time, the kind of treatment and support you have early on can make a big difference to getting back to work successfully.

What causes MSDs at work?

There are many aspects of work that can cause MSDs or make them worse. These include lifting or moving heavy or awkward items (which is referred to as manual handing), doing repetitive tasks that involve making the same movements over and over again, and working at a poorly set up computer (which is often called display screen equipment or visual display unit work because these are the terms used in the regulations).

Because these kinds of risks are common in virtually all workplaces, MSDs can occur in all industries and businesses. They are particularly common in certain jobs like construction, health services and farming, but they also affect people in desk jobs.

What you need to know about MSDs and the law

Your employer has a legal duty to protect your health and safety, and this includes MSDs. As well as the Health and Safety at Work Act 1974, there are several other regulations that are particularly relevant to MSDs at work (see chapter 19).

- The Management of Health and Safety at Work Regulations 1999 require employers to assess the risks to your health and safety via a risk assessment.

- The Manual Handling Operations Regulations 1992 require an employer to carry out a risk assessment on the manual handling tasks that pose a risk of injury.

- There is specific legislation that applies to computer work. These are the Health and Safety (Display Screen Equipment) Regulations 1992. These regulations apply whether you work in an office, at home or are a mobile worker and cover hot-desking as well as fixed workstations. The DSE Regulations mean that employers must do a DSE risk assessment, reduce any risks, provide an eye test if you ask for one, and provide you with the right training and information.

- The Equality Act 2010 protects you from discrimination and requires your employer to provide reasonable adjustments if you have a disability. Many MSDs could be considered a disability under the Act (see Chapters 7 and 15).

- Power tools like hammer drills and chainsaws produce vibration that can damage the nerves, blood vessels and joints in your hands and arms. The Control of Vibration at Work Regulations 2005 require your employer to do a risk assessment and make sure that your exposure to vibration is below a certain limit.

- It's a legal requirement for employers to report ill health at work. RIDDOR (Reporting of Injuries, Diseases and Dangerous

Occurrences Regulations) mean that they must keep accurate records, certain types of ill health must be reported to the HSE, and your employer should encourage you to report injuries and work-related ill health.

Health and Safety Executive www.hse.gov.uk/msd/legislation

Preventing MSDs at work

There is nothing inevitable about MSDs, but because your work can cause MSDs or make them worse, workplaces have a key role to play in preventing MSDs from developing or getting worse. 'For many years there has been a perception that MSK (musculoskeletal) conditions are unavoidable and part of the ageing process,' says Professor Kevin Fenton, Director of health and wellbeing at Public Health England. 'However, most issues can be prevented and the workplace offers a unique opportunity to prevent the development of MSK conditions.'[8]

According to the HSE, the most effective ways of tackling MSDs at work are senior management commitment, worker involvement, risk assessment, controls, training and medical management.[9]

The most important parts of preventing MSDs at work are the way your work – and your workplace – is designed. These factors are the responsibility of employers: it's their legal responsibility to protect your health by using risk assessments and complying with regulations on manual handling, display screen equipment and ill-health reporting (see box).

Once your employers have done a risk assessment, they must tackle any risks they have identified using a hierarchy of controls. The first thing they should do is to eliminate the risk completely, for example by redesigning particular tasks, providing mechanical aids that remove the need for you to lift objects, introducing breaks or job rotation. Because you know the most about risks associated with your work, your employer should always consult you and your trade union when doing risk assessments. They should also monitor the changes they've made to ensure they are working effectively.

Having the correct training is an important way of reducing the risk of workplace MSDs, and the law says that your employer must train you to use equipment correctly (see box). This kind of training should include things like good handling and moving techniques, using equipment, reporting injuries and how to spot and avoid dangers.[10]

There are also ways that you can help protect yourself at work. Your employer should give you proper breaks, but you should ensure that you take these. This will help reduce the risks of MSDs that are associated with repetitive work. Use your break to use different muscles, for example by getting up, stretching and walking around if you've been sitting at a computer. If you do finding any work tasks painful, it's important to tell your employer and your union rep as soon as possible.[11]

Reducing your risk

Assuming that your employer is doing everything they can – and should – to remove the risks associated with MSDs at work, your lifestyle will also have an impact on MSDs. As well as your age, your levels of activity and strength will affect your risk of developing MSDs. Less obvious things will make a difference too, such as your weight, your diet and whether you smoke. These things are also interconnected. For example, two risk factors that often coincide are age and activity, because we tend to be less active as we get older. Whereas three-quarters of people aged 19–24 are physically active, that's true of only 25% of people over 85 years old.[12]

Public Health England's advice is that adults should aim to take at least 150 minutes of moderate intensity physical activity a week in bouts of at least 10 minutes. In 2017, they launched a simple mobile phone app called Active 10 to encourage you to hit these targets.

As well as being active daily, you should spend less time being sedentary and do something to improve your muscle strength on at least two days a week. This needn't involved going to the gym, it could be carrying heavy shopping or doing yoga where you are supporting your own body weight, and it's important because it reduces the risk of losing muscle mass.

Maintaining a healthy weight can also reduce the risks of developing MSDs such as back pain and osteoarthritis of the knee. When researchers looked at evidence from 47 studies involving more than 466,000 people, they found a three-fold increased risk in the development of knee OA in overweight or obese individuals.[13] Healthy bones also depend on having a healthy diet, and in particular on how much calcium and vitamin D you get. There is vitamin D in some foods, but it's difficult for us to get enough vitamin D from food alone and our main source of vitamin D comes from the action of sunlight on our skin.

Our bodies make vitamin D when our skin is exposed to sunlight. If you don't absorb much sunlight, either because you work indoors, or have dark skin, always cover your skin. Public Health England advice is to consider taking a vitamin D supplement of 10 micrograms a day all year. Even if you do get outside, the UK's latitude means that during autumn and winter the sun isn't strong enough for our bodies to make enough vitamin D, so everyone should consider taking a vitamin D supplement between October and the end of March.[14]

Smoking is associated with many diseases, from cancer to cardiovascular disease, but it's also bad for bone density. Public Health England looked at scientific studies of smoking and bone health and found that smoking is associated with several MSDs.

For example, smokers have 60% more back, neck and leg pain and are more than twice as likely to have such bad back pain that it's disabling.

Smoking has more impact on reduced bone density in post-menopausal women (see chapter 18), is associated with bone fractures and slower healing of fractures, is a significant cause of rheumatoid arthritis and can make treatment less effective.[15]

We saw earlier that having a MSD can increase your risk of developing depression, and the reverse is also true. People with depression are at greater risk of developing back pain, so there is a vicious circle involving mental health and the pain and disability associated with MSDs.

CASE STUDY MSDs, ageing and work

Employers need to make sure they are complying with health and safety laws, but because – and despite the fact that – MSDs are so common, much more research is needed to find better ways to manage and prevent MSDs at work.

In 2014, Arthritis UK and the Medical Research Council provided funding to set up a new Centre for Musculoskeletal Health and Work at the University of Southampton. The centre's research focuses on back, neck and arm pain – the three main causes of work disability. Their projects include looking at whether using social media and online campaigns to spread information about managing back pain works, and developing new guidelines for people with osteoarthritis and carpal tunnel syndrome so that employers can plan their return to work properly.

They are also particularly interested in how MSDs affect older workers. Andy Briggs, CEO of Aviva UK Life and the government's Business Champion for Older Workers, wants to see one million more older people in work by 2022. Achieving this depends on paying much more attention to MSDs among older workers.[16]

To do this, the Centre for Musculoskeletal Health and Work has established a study called Health and Employment After 50 (HEAF), which is following a group of 8,000 people aged between 50 and 64 using annual questionnaires about work and health. HEAF has already found that MSDs are among the commonest health reasons for people in this age group leaving work.[17]

Researchers are also using HEAF data to study frailty, which includes symptoms like exhaustion, slow walking speed and poor grip strength. Frailty has a major impact on how long people are able to keep working, and the researchers want to find ways of screening older workers so that they can support those who are most likely to struggle to remain in work (see chapter 8).

Arthritis UK www.arthritisresearchuk.org/news/press-releases/2014/november/work-centre.aspx

Treating MSDs – and returning to work

As well as taking proactive approach to preventing MSDs, there are several other actions your employer should take if you develop a MSD and have to take time off work. Because treatment is likely to be most effective the earlier it begins, it's important to report MSDs as soon as you think there is a problem. This will also allow your employer to tackle the causes by adjusting your work. And if you have access to an occupational health service at work, they will have a key role to play.

If you do have to take a significant amount of time off work, then your employer should also manage your return to work in a coordinated way. This includes agreeing a return to work plan with you and your doctor, gradually building up your hours in what's called a 'phased return to work', and making adjustments to your hours and tasks. They should also bear in mind that MSDs can have a significant impact on people's mental health, so that as well as dealing with physical and occupational issues, your employer should also address any psychological factors.[18]

Notes

1 HSE (2017) *Work-related Musculoskeletal Disorders (WRMSDs) Statistics in Great Britain 2017*. www.hse.gov.uk/statistics/ causdis/musculoskeletal/msd.pdf

2 ONS (2017) www.ons.gov.uk/news/news/ totalof137millionworkingdayslosttosicknessandinjuryin2016

3 HSE (2017) *Work-related Musculoskeletal Disorders (WRMSDs) statistics in Great Britain 2017*. www.hse.gov.uk/statistics/causdis/ musculoskeletal/msd.pdf

4 Public Health England (2017) *Productive healthy ageing and musculoskeletal (MSK) health*. www.gov.uk/government/ publications/productive-healthy-ageing-and-musculoskeletal-health/productive-healthy-ageing-and-musculoskeletal-msk-health

5 ETUC (2016) *The pain that's crippling Europe*. www.etuc.org/ press/pain-thats-crippling-europe#.WsSobpPwZE6

6 Public Health England (2017) *Productive healthy ageing and musculoskeletal (MSK) health*. www.gov.uk/government/ publications/productive-healthy-ageing-and-musculoskeletal-health/productive-healthy-ageing-and-musculoskeletal-msk-health

7 Fit for Work (2015) https://fitforwork.org/blog/musculoskeletal-disorders-msds-and-depression/

8 Business in the Community (2017) *Musculoskeletal health in the workplace: a toolkit for employers*. https://wellbeing.bitc.org.uk/ sites/default/files/business_in_the_community_musculoskeletal_ toolkit.pdf

9 www.hse.gov.uk/msd/faq-general.htm

10 UNISON www.unison.org.uk/get-help/knowledge/health-and-safety/back-pain

11 Fit for Work (2016) https://fitforwork.org/blog/musculoskeletal-disorders-and-manual-jobs/

12 Public Health England (2017) Productive healthy ageing and musculoskeletal (MSK) health. www.gov.uk/government/publications/productive-healthy-ageing-and-musculoskeletal-health/productive-healthy-ageing-and-musculoskeletal-msk-health

13 Muthuri, SG et al. (2011) What if we prevent obesity? Risk reduction in knee osteoarthritis estimated through a meta-analysis of observational studies. *Arthritis Care & Research*, **63**, 7, pp. 982–990 (July). https://onlinelibrary.wiley.com/doi/epdf/10.1002/acr.20464

14 Scientific Advisory Committee on Nutrition (2016) *Vitamin D and health*. www.gov.uk/government/publications/sacn-vitamin-d-and-health-report

15 Public Health England (2014) *Smoking: progressive decline of the body's major systems*. www.gov.uk/government/publications/smoking-progressive-decline-of-the-bodys-major-systems

16 http://worklife-blog.org/tag/health-and-employment-after-fifty-heaf-study

17 www.arthritisresearchuk.org/news/arthritis-today/2017/august/can-we-really-work-for-longer.aspx

18 BITC (2017) *Musculoskeletal health in the workplace*. www.hse.gov.uk/sicknessabsence/msd.htm

Chapter 7
Disability discrimination and reasonable adjustments

One in two adults of working age with a disability are in employment, against an overall UK employment rate of 75%. With one in six working age adults reporting that they have a disability, the impact is significant, which led the government to publish a new strategy in late 2017[1] for improving the opportunities of people with disabilities and long-term health problems to find, remain and thrive in work. This will see changes in the welfare system, health services and at the workplace. The government has also set a target of 4.5 million disabled people in work by 2027, which would implement the Conservative Party's 2017 general election manifesto promise of one million more disabled people in work than in 2017.

Tackling discrimination

The Equality Act 2010 protects individuals with disabilities against discrimination or detriment as a result of their disability, which is defined as a physical or mental impairment that 'has a substantial and long-term adverse effect' (12 months in practice) on the person's ability to carry out normal day-to-day activities. If you have cancer, HIV or multiple sclerosis, for example, you are protected from when you are diagnosed. The Equalities and Human Rights Commission publishes advice for employees on the Equality Act, [2] and the TUC's website offers helpful guidance on disability discrimination at work.

The Equality Act covers six types of disability discrimination that may apply in the context of work:

- direct discrimination – your employer treats you worse than another person in a similar situation because of your disability;

- indirect discrimination – your employer has a policy or procedure that has a worse impact on disabled people than on people who are not disabled;

- failure to make reasonable adjustments (see later in this chapter);

- discrimination arising from disability – you are treated badly because of a disability-related issue, for example needing time off for medical appointments;

- harassment – someone makes you feel humiliated, offended or degraded; and

- victimization – you are treated badly because you have made a complaint of discrimination under the Equality Act.

The Act says that employers cannot ask job applicants about their health or disability until they have been offered a job, except in specific circumstances where the information is necessary for the application process or a requirement of the job.

Applying for a job

The Act covers situations in which you are applying for a job. The EHRC emphasizes that employers can only ask job applicants questions about your health or any disability 'in very restricted circumstances or for very restricted purposes', until you have been offered a job or included in a pool of successful candidates to be offered a job'.[3] It is legitimate, however, for a prospective employer to ask you some questions at an early stage to establish whether it needs to make reasonable adjustments for you to undergo an assessment, whether you will be able to carry out functions that are intrinsic to the job, for monitoring functions, or if it needs someone with a specific disability to do the job.[4]

It is lawful for an offer of a job to be conditional on your passing an occupational health check, with the government Equalities Office advising that if the check shows that your disability affects your ability to do the job:

> The question will then be whether a reasonable adjustment can be made to deal with that. If a reasonable adjustment cannot be made, it would then be legitimate to withdraw the job offer on the grounds that the applicant has not met the required condition.[5]

Reasonable adjustments

If you qualify as a disabled person under the Act, your employer must make reasonable adjustments to any elements of your job that place you at a substantial disadvantage compared to persons who are not disabled. The duty relates to:

- a provision, criterion or practice applied by or on behalf of your employer, for example a requirement by your employer that people who do your job to work full time and for fixed hours;

- a physical feature of your employer's premises, for example, if steps to a building prevented access by a person in a wheelchair or the toilets were inaccessible to a person; and

- the lack of an auxiliary aid or service, for example a signer or reader.

It is important to remember that your employer need only make the adjustment if it is reasonable. The judgement as to what is reasonable will depend on factors such as cost, practicability, your employer's resources and size, and how effective the adjustment is likely to prove.

There are numerous examples of what might constitute a reasonable adjustment. Below, we list some examples, drawn mainly from the EHRC and the government Equalities Office:

- making adjustments to premises, such as widening a door or a ramp for a wheelchair user, or providing appropriate contrast in decor to help a visually impaired person;

- allocating some of your duties to another person, either temporarily or permanently;

- if there are no reasonable adjustments that would allow you to continue in your current job, transferring you to an existing vacancy;

- altering your hours of work so that you do not have to travel in the rush hour;

- mentoring, for example if you have returned to work after a lengthy absence;

- acquiring or modifying equipment, for example a large screen for a visually impaired person or an adapted keyboard for a person with arthritis;

- offering training, for example in the use of equipment that will help you do your job or where you need training to operate equipment used by your colleagues;

- allowing you to be absent during working hours for rehabilitation, assessment or medical treatment;
- providing instructions for equipment in braille or an audible means (for example on a CD or via a smartphone);
- allowing a guide dog or hearing dog into the workplace;
- providing additional supervisory guidance and support;
- including a disabled car parking space.

Your employer must also ensure that your colleagues cooperate when making a reasonable adjustment. For example, a reasonable adjustment for a person with autism might be to have a highly structured day, which might prove unpopular with some other workers. The EHRC advises that it would be unlikely that your employer could successfully argue that an adjustment was unreasonable because other staff were obstructive or unhelpful when it attempted the adjustment.

Guidance from the EHRC[6] is clear that in particular, if you are a disabled person, the need to make adjustments for you as a worker or job applicant:

- must not be a reason not to appoint you to a job or promote you if you are the best person for the job with the adjustments in place;
- must be considered in relation to every aspect of your job provided the adjustments are reasonable for the employer to make.

Mental health adjustments

Most of the adjustments suggested above are most relevant to physical disabilities. The Act, however, also covers mental impairments. Reasonable adjustments here may include adjusting the workload or pace of work, including allowing different start and finish times to the working day and discounting disability-related sickness leave for the purposes of absence management.

The Department of Health (DoH) has produced some practical prompts for employees and their line managers to explore when considering workplace adjustments for disabled persons with mental health problems. These cover working hours or patterns, the physical environment, support with workload and support from others (see 'Prompts' box).[7] 'Being flexible and creative,' the DoH adds, 'is important when considering solutions.' The EHRC[8] has also published advice that contains examples of adjustments, including for depression and autism (see page 93).

Mental health adjustment 'Prompts'

The Department of Health suggests the following prompts when considering reasonable adjustments for persons with mental health problems:

Working hours or patterns

- Take a flexible approach to start/finish times and/or shift patterns.
- Allow use of paid or unpaid leave for medical appointments.
- Phase the return to work, for example by offering temporary part-time hours.
- Equal amount of break time, but in shorter, more frequent chunks.
- Allow someone to arrange their annual leave so that is spaced regularly throughout the year.
- Allow the possibility to work from home at times.
- Temporary reallocation of some tasks.

Physical environment

- Minimize noise – for example, providing private office/room dividers/partitions, reducing pitch or volume of telephone ring tones.
- Provide a quiet space for breaks away from the main workspace.
- Offer a reserved parking space.
- Allow for increased personal space.
- Move the workstation – to ensure for example that someone does not have their back to the door.

Support with workload

- Increase frequency of supervision.
- Support someone to prioritize their work.
- Allow the individual to focus on a specific piece of work.
- Consider job sharing.

Support from others

- Provide a job coach.
- Provide a buddy or mentor.
- Provide mediation if there are difficulties between colleagues.

Remedies

If you think your employer or a prospective employer has failed to make a reasonable adjustment, you should ask for an explanation and involve your union or staff representative, if you have one, and consider complaining to your employer. If you cannot resolve the situation, you can lodge a claim for unlawful discrimination under the Act with the Employment Tribunal.

From the date on which you believe you suffered discrimination, you have three months, less one day, in which to complain to the tribunal.

Before you do this, however, you will have to go through the Early Conciliation Procedure, under which you submit an early conciliation form[9] to Acas, or telephone Acas with your details and those of your employer. Acas will offer a free conciliation service to try to resolve the dispute. The three-month time limit will usually be extended pending the conciliation process.

If you are successful, the Employment Tribunal can declare your employer has discriminated against you, award you compensation (for financial losses such as loss of earnings) and damages for injury to your feelings, and make a recommendation that your employer do something specific to correct the situation or remove the bad effects, for example by reinstating you. Further details on Employment Tribunals are contained in the final chapter of this book, on realising your rights.

Reasonable adjustments for depression and autism

The Equalities and Human Rights Commission suggests the following reasonable adjustments for persons with depression and autism.[10]

Depression

A worker's performance has recently got worse and they have started being late for work. Previously they had a very good record of punctuality and performance. Rather than just telling them they must improve, their employer talks to them in private. This allows the employer to check whether the change in performance could be for a disability-related reason. The worker says that they are experiencing a recurrence of depression and are not sleeping well which is making them late. Together the employer and the worker agree to change the worker's hours slightly while they are in this situation and that the worker can ask for help whenever they are finding it difficult to start or complete a task. These are reasonable adjustments.

Autism

An employer makes sure that a worker with autism has a structured working day as a reasonable adjustment. As part of the reasonable adjustment, it is the responsibility of the employer to make sure that other workers co-operate with this arrangement.

Access to work

As we noted in our chapter on mental health, the government's Access to Work scheme[11] may be able to give you a grant to help you start, remain in or return to, work – particularly in circumstances where your needs may be adjustments that might not be deemed reasonable for your employer to make. Access to Work is available to individuals who are disabled or have a mental or physical health condition that affects their paid work. After you have applied, an Access to Work adviser will contact you to discuss the possible assistance. The adviser may visit your workplace to determine your needs and contact your employer but will only do so after first having spoken to you. Potential support includes:

- British Sign Language interpreters and video relay service support, lip speakers or note takers;

- a support worker or job coach to help you in your workplace;

- a support service, such as counselling, if you have a mental health condition;

- disability awareness training for your colleagues;

- the cost of moving your equipment if you change location; and

- help getting to and from work (including, adaptations of your vehicle, taxi fares or a support worker if you cannot use public transport).

Further help

Equality and Human Rights Commission, www.equalityhumanrights.com/en, tel: 0808 800 0082

The Equality Advisory Support Service (EASS) provides advice on discrimination issues and legal rights and remedies: bit.ly/2vHVGyo; tel: 0808 800 0082

Access to Work, www.gov.uk/access-to-work

TUC: www.tuc.org.uk and www.stuc.org.uk, tel: 020 7636 4030

Disability Rights UK: www.disabilityrightsuk.org

Acas (The Independent Advisory, Conciliation and Arbitration Service): www.acas.org.uk, tel: 08457 474747

Acas Helpline: 0300 123 1100

Employment Tribunal Service: www.gov.uk/courts-tribunals/ employment-tribunal. Enquiry Line: 0300 123 1024 (England and Wales) or 0141 354 8574 (Scotland)

Disability Law Service (DLS), which provides information and advice to disabled and deaf people: www.dls.org.uk, tel: 020 7791 9800

Association of Disabled Professionals, which offers advice, support, resources and general information for disabled professionals, entrepreneurs and employers: www.adp.org.uk, tel: 01204 431638

Government Equalities Office: www.gov.uk/government/organisations/government-equalities-office, tel: 020 7211 6000

Citizens Advice, which was formerly known as Citizens Advice Bureau, is a network of over 300 independent charities that offer advice on a range of issues, including employment. Your local Citizens Advice may be able to put you in touch with a specialist lawyer: www.citizensadvice.org.uk/work/health-and-safety-at-work/accidents-at-work-overview

Law centres can offer legal advice, casework and representation to individuals who cannot afford a lawyer: www.lawcentres.org.uk/i-am-looking-for-advice, tel: 0203 637 1330. Check with the Law Centres Network whether there is a centre that covers the area where you live: www.lawcentres.org.uk/about-law-centres/law-centres-on-google-maps/alphabetically

The LawWorks Clinics Network provides free initial advice to individuals on various areas including employment law. It operates in England and Wales and will put you in touch with volunteer lawyers, if you are not eligible for legal aid and cannot afford to pay for legal help. To find a clinic near you: www.lawworks.org.uk/legal-advice-individuals/find-legal-advice-clinic-near-you

AdviceUK has 700 members and advises a further 500 organizations. Although it will not advise you directly, you can use its website to find your nearest advice centre: www.adviceuk.org.uk/looking-for-advice/find-advice

Health and Safety Executive: www.hse.gov.uk, tel: 08701 545 500

Notes

1 Department for Work and Pensions, Department of Health (2017), *Improving lives. The future of work, health and disability*. Cm 9526, assets.publishing.service.gov.uk/government/uploads/system/uploads/attachment_data/file/663400/print-ready-improving-lives-the-future-of-work-health-and-disability.pdf

2 www.equalityhumanrights.com/en/advice-and-guidance/equality-act-guidance#h2

3 EHRC (2014) *Your rights to equality at work: when you apply for a job*, www.equalityhumanrights.com/sites/default/files/your_rights_to_equality_at_work_-_applying_for_a_job.pdf

4 EHRC (2014) *Pre-employment health questions: guidance for job applications on Section 60 of the Equality Act 2010*, www.equalityhumanrights.com/sites/default/files/pre-employment_health_questions_for_job_applicants_0.pdf

5 Government Equalities Office, Equality Act 2010. Duty on employers to make reasonable adjustments for their staff, bit.ly/2poOUYa

6 EHRC (2014) *Your rights to equality at work: when you apply for a job*, www.equalityhumanrights.com/sites/default/files/your_rights_to_equality_at_work_-_applying_for_a_job.pdf

7 Department of Health, *Advice for employers on workplace adjustments for mental health conditions*, www.nhshealthatwork.co.uk/images/library/files/government%20policy/Mental_Health_Adjustments_Guidance_May_2012.pdf

8 www.equalityhumanrights.com/en/multipage-guide/employment-workplace-adjustments

9 Guidance on the early conciliation procedure and a notification form is available at www.ec.acas.org.uk

10 www.equalityhumanrights.com/en/multipage-guide/employment-workplace-adjustments

11 www.gov.uk/access-to-work

Chapter 8
An ageing workforce

In 2018, the number of over-50s in the UK workforce topped 10 million for the first time. We often hear that the workforce is ageing, both as a result of changes in the population and changes in legislation. Despite this, myths and stereotypes abound. We need to untangle the facts about health, work and age so that we can make workplaces more age-friendly.

Work, age and health

Throughout our lives, health and work are intimately intertwined; our health affects our work and our work affects our health. Health in older age partly depends on the cumulative effects of lifestyle, environmental and workplace exposures. Given that we spend a significant proportion of our lives at work, safe and healthy workplaces make a big difference to our overall physical and mental health.

So does being without work. Being unemployed has negative effects on physical and mental health, and there are differences in mortality rates between people in managerial jobs compared with those in less skilled jobs. For example, almost 20% of male manual workers die before reaching State Pension Age, compared with 7% of men in higher social classes. As well as living on average four years less, male and female manual workers also have higher rates of ill health in retirement.[1]

Good work, however, can bring many health benefits, and vice versa. Staying healthy affects how long you're likely to be able to continue working and for many of us, work is a source of self-worth and companionship as well as a source of income. And while poor jobs can expose to you to hazards that damage your health – such as noise, chemicals and long hours – good workplaces can help you lead a healthier lifestyle (see chapter 11).

The UK's workforce is ageing. But before looking at what that means for your health at work, we need to unpack some common attitudes to age. We'll discover that it's often the myths and stereotypes surrounding older workers that prevent people working into older age if they want to. We'll also see that there are many simple things that you and your employer can do to remove those barriers. But first, we need to consider what we mean by terms such as 'old' and 'older', and how useful they are at work.

Am I old?

Whether you are considered 'old' depends on many things, including where you live and who you ask. The United Nations, for example, describes you as 'older' when you reach 60, but 'older' is a relative term. Sixty probably still seems relatively young in Japan, for example, where people live the longest (women's life expectancy is 86.8 years in Japan), but in Sierra Leone, average life expectancy is just 50.8 for women and 49.3 for men.[2]

As well as making a major difference to life expectancy between nations, inequality has a big impact on life expectancy within countries. The latest data from the Office for National Statistics show that for boys born in England between 2012 and 2014, the richest will live almost a decade longer than the poorest.[3]

Attitudes to age also differ depending on who you ask. A European Union survey of more than 26,000 people across 27 EU Member States found that the average age at which you start to be considered 'old' is 63.9. People in the Netherlands say you're old when you reach 70, but if you live in Slovakia, you're considered old at 57.7 years. The survey also revealed how much your own age influences your perceptions of other people's age. It found that 15–24-year-olds think old age begins around 59, but if you're over 55, you think old age doesn't begin until you're 67.[4]

Lastly and most importantly, ageing is an individual process and all older workers are different. You'll probably have 70-year-old friends who are fitter than some 30-year-olds that you know. That's because ageing is a biological process influenced by many factors. Your biological age is not the same as chronological age. How old you are simply depends on how many years you've been alive, while biological age – which has a big impact on your health – depends on other things, including your genes, your parents' health, your environmental or workplace exposures, and lifestyle factors such as smoking, diet, alcohol consumption and physical activity.

This means that chronological age isn't the best predictor of health, and ageing is not inevitably linked to illness and disease. It also means that at work, age is not a terribly useful indicator of how well you can do your job. Rather than your age in years, the European Agency for Safety and Health at Work recommends focusing on your 'work ability' – ie, what you need depending on the demands of your work.[5] And in the future, it's possible that we might find ways of measuring people's biological age rather than their chronological age.[6]

Busting myths and challenging stereotypes

Even though the workforce is ageing, there are many persistent myths and negative stereotypes about older workers. People might assume that older workers are more likely to suffer from certain health conditions, that they have more time off sick, that they're slower, more stuck in their ways and less able to learn new things. We all need to challenge these stereotypes because they are untrue and can result in discrimination.

In fact, the evidence shows that when it comes to sickness absence, for example, older workers don't take more sick leave than younger workers. Instead, patterns of absence vary with age. In general, younger workers have more short-term sickness absence while older workers have more longer-term sick leave. And although many people assume that workers' physical health declines because of chronic diseases like heart trouble or musculoskeletal problems due to heavy manual work, the data shows that most older workers have good health and are certainly well enough to do their jobs well into their late 60s.[7]

These negative stereotypes tend to be more prominent than the positive attributes of older workers. Your age and experience are valuable assets to employers. According to a government survey of almost 700 private-sector employers in the UK, experience, reliability and the ability to mentor younger staff were cited as the most important benefits of having workers aged 50 or over in their organizations.[8] And being part of an age-diverse workforce brings other benefits to workplaces, from new ideas and better problem solving to a better understanding of the needs of older customers.[9]

Interestingly, we don't know much about health and safety in workers over the age of 65 because very few studies have been done. This is a gap in our knowledge that the Health and Safety Laboratory has flagged up.[10]

Challenging stereotypes

If you want to challenge stereotypes about older workers, you're not alone and there are plenty of resources to draw on. The World Health Organization's new global strategy on healthy ageing aims to create age-friendly environments by changing to the way we think about older people.

The WHO strategy stresses that 'every older person is different' and that health is crucial to how we experience older age – in the workplace and in our communities. During its 'Decade of Healthy Ageing' from 2020 to 2030, the WHO will be mounting a global campaign to combat ageism.

To find out more, visit www.who.int/ageing/en and follow #yearsahead on Twitter.

An ageing population and ageing workforce

The make-up of the world's population is changing rapidly and in far-reaching ways. People are living longer and birth rates are lower than they were in the past. This means that the world's population is ageing, shifting the balance between younger and older people.[11] The same is true in the UK. There are more older people in the population and older people make up a growing proportion of the population. The UK's population structure today is very different from what it was in the past. For example, over-65s made up around 18% of the UK population in 2014, a rise of 47% since 1974.[12] This trend is set to continue and by 2024, more than one in four people in the UK will be over 60.[13]

The UK workforce is also ageing. This is because that together with increased life expectancy, there have been important changes in retirement laws and the age at which you can claim your state pension. The UK default retirement age was abolished in 2011, and State Pension Age (SPA) is rising. From 2020, SPA for men and women will be 66; this will increase to 67 between 2026 and 2028, after which SPA will be linked to life expectancy. It remains to be seen how Brexit affects the UK workforce through reduced migration and mobility of labour.

In 2016, there were more than 1.2 million people working over the age of 65, and in 2018 the number of over 50s in the UK workforce topped 10 million for the first time. That means that almost one-third of the UK workforce is over 50, compared with one in five in the early 1990s.

All this has profound effects, both on older workers and employers. From an individual point of view, people will need to work for longer in order to afford longer retirements. And if employers are to avoid labour shortages, they will need to do much more to recruit and retain more older workers.

Several organizations, such as Business in the Community (BITC) and the Centre for Ageing Better, have warned employers and the government that they need to do more to support older workers. Many older people without jobs want to work, says BITC. They estimate that 1.2 million people in the UK aged over 50 would be willing to work given the right conditions, and between 2017 and 2022 BITC want to see 1 million more people over the age of 50 in fulfilling work.[14]

Championing older workers

When the number of over 50s in the UK workforce topped 10 million for the first time in 2018, the Centre for Ageing Better (CfAB) called on employers and the government to make sure that employment practices provide better support to older workers.

Helping more older workers stay in work is vital for the economy and for individuals, yet there are around one million older people in the UK who want to work but are not in work. Nearly half of 50–60 year-olds have a long-term health condition, and health is the single biggest reason why people leave the workforce.[15]

The CfAB argue that:

- Employers need to realize that older workers are valuable.

- Working practices need to include older workers rather than disadvantage them.

- Adjustments need to be made to workplaces, from allowing flexible working and tackling ageism in recruitment to making sure older workers have equal access to training and career progression.

Health and older workers

Given that people will need to work for longer, what do we know about the health and safety of older workers? And is it health or other things that are preventing people from staying in – or re-entering – the workforce if they want to?

The British Medical Association has reviewed the evidence on how our health changes as we age and what impact – if any – this has on work:[16]

- They looked at dozens of studies including data on age-related hearing loss, eyesight, aerobic capacity and muscle strength, diseases such as cancer and heart disease as well as mental health, menopause (see chapter 18) and prostate problems. They also looked at whether age affects workplace accident rates and shift work.

- Even though hearing, strength and other functional abilities decline with age, this varies a great deal from one person and another and has a minimal impact on working-age people. The incidence of cancer, heart disease, arthritis and other long-term conditions increase with age but have very little impact on job performance. And as far as work-related accidents and ill health are concerned, it's your occupation rather than your age that matters most.

• Overall, people with long-term conditions manage to work, and declining health has very little impact on performance and safety in most jobs. Also, if certain things become difficult, older workers often draw on their experience to find other ways of doing them.

Your rights at work

• The Equality Act 2010 makes it unlawful for your employer to discriminate against you because of your age.

• Since 2011, your employer can't automatically force you to retire once you reach the state pension age. That means you can usually work for as long as want, unless your employer has a good reason, for example because your job requires certain physical capabilities or has a legal age limit set by law, such as the fire service.

• You have a legal right to request flexible working, provided you have worked for the same employer for 26 weeks. Your employer must handle your request in a reasonable manner, but if they have a good business reason, they can refuse your request.

• Health and safety should not be used as an excuse not to employ older people.

Creating age-friendly workplaces

Creating age-friendly workplaces isn't difficult. By understanding more about ageing, work and health and consulting – rather than making assumptions about – older workers, workplaces can be made healthier for everyone. And while what is good for older workers will be good for younger ones too, surveys of older workers show that flexible working is really important.

Flexible working is key to making work more age-friendly, and you have the right to request flexible working (see previous box). Flexible working means a range of things, such as reduced hours, part-time working and being able to work from home. This flexibility makes it easier for you to combine work with managing your own health and caring responsibilities. Find out whether your workplace has a flexible working champion and speak to your trade union rep. Acas has a free booklet aimed at employees and employers on flexible working and work-life balance.[17]

Employers must conduct risk assessments – this is a legal duty under the Management of Health and Safety at Work Regulations 1999 (see chapter 19). Risk assessments enable employers to identify and minimize risks. Although a separate risk assessment isn't required for older workers, the HSE says that employers should think about activities that older workers do so that they can make changes if necessary.[18]

Your job can also be redesigned to fit in with your health conditions. This might include changing what your job involves, for example making your job more varied, giving you more control over it, and using all the experience you've built up. It might mean adjusting the pace and volume of your work, your deadlines and any physical strain. It could also mean changing the kind of work you do. Or it might mean providing certain equipment, such as better lighting or bigger computer screens.

Your occupational health and safety service will be really useful, and the work they do helps everyone, not only older workers (see chapter 12). In fact, by adopting healthier lifestyles sooner, your younger colleagues will benefit the most from workplace health promotion (see chapter 11). Your trade union safety representatives, if you have them, are also important. They help ensure that all workers have a safe and healthy workplace, so make it more likely that older people will be able to enjoy a long and illness-free old age.

The Department for Work and Pensions has produced a useful collection of case studies – real examples of older workers in a range of different jobs – to illustrate how employers are responding to an ageing workforce[19] – and the National Centre for Sport & Exercise Medicine East Midlands has developed a free online course on the benefits of physical activity for older adults.[20]

Notes

1 TUC (2014) *The health and safety of older workers*. www.tuc. org.uk/research-analysis/reports/national/health-and-safety-older-workers-guidance

2 WHO. *Global Health Observatory data*. www.who.int/gho/mortality_burden_disease/life_tables/situation_trends/en/

3 ONS (2018) *Health state life expectancies by national deprivation deciles, England and Wales: 2014 to 2016*. www.ons.gov.uk/peoplepopulationandcommunity/healthandsocialcare/healthinequalities/bulletins/healthstatelifeexpectanciesbyindexofmultipledeprivationimd/englandandwales2014to2016

4 European Commission (2012) *Special Eurobarometer 378: Active Ageing*. https://ec.europa.eu/eip/ageing/library/special-eurobarometer-378-active-ageing_en

5 EU-OSHA (2016) The ageing workforce: Implications for occupational safety and health. A research review. https://osha.europa.eu/sites/default/files/publications/documents/the-ageing-workforce-implications-for-occupational-safety-and-health-a-research-review-executive-summary.pdf

6 UK Parliament (2018) *The Ageing Process and Health POST Note*. https://researchbriefings.parliament.uk/ResearchBriefing/Summary/POST-PN-0571

7 BMA (2016) *Ageing and the workplace.* www.bma.org.uk/advice/employment/occupational-health/ageing-and-the-workplace

8 DWP (2015) *Employer attitudes to fuller working lives.* www.gov.uk/government/uploads/system/uploads/attachment_data/file/410660/employer-attitudes-to-fuller-working-lives.pdf

9 Acas. *Age and the workplace.* www.acas.org.uk/media/pdf/e/4/Age-and-the-workplace-guide.pdf. How an ageing workforce can revitalise your business www.acas.org.uk/index.aspx?articleid=5919

10 HSL. *Working beyond 65: the health and safety impact.* www.hsl.gov.uk/resources/health-safety-insights/working-beyond-65-the-health-and-safety-impact

11 BMA (2016) *Ageing and the workplace*

12 Ibid.

13 ONS (2016) *How the population of England is projected to age.* www.ons.gov.uk/peoplepopulationandcommunity/populationandmigration/populationprojections/compendium/subnationalpopulationprojectionssupplementaryanalysis/2014basedprojections/howthepopulationofenglandisprojectedtoage

14 BITC (2014) *The missing million.* https://age.bitc.org.uk/all-resources/research-articles/missing-million-report-1

15 Centre for Ageing Better (2017) *What do older workers value about work and why?* www.ageing-better.org.uk/publications/fulfilling-work-what-do-older-workers-value-about-work-and-why

16 BMA (2016) *Ageing and the workplace.*

17 Acas. *Flexible working and work-life balance.* www.acas.org.uk/media/pdf/3/1/Flexible_working_and_work_life_balance_Nov.pdf

18 HSE. *Health and safety for older workers.* www.hse.gov.uk/vulnerable-workers/older-workers.htm

19 DWP (2011) *Employer case studies: Employing older workers for an effective multi-generational workforce*. www.gov.uk/ government/uploads/system/uploads/attachment_data/file/142752/ employing-older-workers-case-studies.pdf

20 NCSEM-EM (2017) www.ncsem-em.org.uk/research/ncsem-em-launches-older-adults-resource-with-public-health-england

Chapter 9
Working time

You will likely have come across reports of academic and medical studies that point to worrying links between long working hours and ill health. The concerns include strokes and cardiovascular diseases, stress and mental ill health, as well as musculoskeletal disorders and possible links to lowered immunity and diabetes.

Many of these studies, however, have limitations. They may, for example: be restricted to one industry or type of work; focus on shift work, night work or unsociable working hours rather than long hours; be unable to rule out other factors that might have contributed to the findings, including lifestyle; have different understandings of how many hours constitute 'long' (usually 48 or 55); or be unable to prove that the ill health is a direct result of working long hours.

In this chapter, we touch on the main concerns by briefly drawing on three reviews that looked at a large number of research studies. There is no doubt that long working hours are associated with many ill-health conditions, although the precise causal mechanisms are usually unclear. The more research that is carried out, however, the more the pieces in the jigsaw fit together, with issues of choice and control over work and work hours and rest breaks, the type of job and the culture of the work environment all playing roles.

In 2015, *The Lancet* published an important review of 25 studies[1] that found an association between long working hours and the risk of a stroke or, to a more modest extent, developing heart disease. The studies covered 600,000 individuals in 11 countries who did not have heart problems at the start of the studies.

The definition of long working hours in the studies was mostly 55 hours or more, though some used 45 hours or more.

The researchers found that people who worked 55 or more hours a week had, compared with those who worked 35–40 hours a week, an increased relative risk of:

- a stroke (increased risk of 33%), with the risk rising as the number of hours worked increased. (People working for 49–54 hours had an increased risk of 27%, while the 10% increased risk for those working 41–48 hours was non-significant);

- heart disease (increased risk of 13%), with the risk higher among those of low socio-economic groups compared with intermediate groups. In the high socioeconomic group, there was no significant link.

In a 2003 research review carried out for the government,[2] the Institute for Employment Studies (IES) noted there was evidence showing associations between long hours of working and health outcomes, such as mental health and cardiovascular problems, and that UK case studies indicated a link between long working hours and minor ill-health problems, particularly among non-manual workers. There were also 'clear grounds' for concern about possible adverse effects of long hours on the frequency of health and safety incidents. The IES also found that long hours working, especially if accompanied by sleep disruption, affected the rate of errors.

The impact of long hours on safety and accidents was picked up in the same year by a review of research from the HSE's Health and Safety Laboratory (HSL), which found that the evidence was 'not conclusive' but that there again seemed to be 'cause for concern', particularly for drivers. The HSL did, however, find an association between working long hours and fatigue, with the effects likely to be 'mediated' by age, sleep, fatigue, experience and a lack of training.

The HSL also concluded there was sufficient evidence for 'concern about the potentially negative effects of working long hours on physical health', with the strongest evidence 'probably' being links to cardiovascular disorder.[3] There was evidence that working long hours could lead to stress or mental ill health, although this was 'somewhat equivocal' and affected by the way in which workers think about their jobs and the amount of control they have over their job (see Chapter 2). From the available evidence, the HSL believed there was 'sufficient reason to be concerned about a possible link between long hours and physical health outcomes, especially for hours exceeding 48–50 per week.' Subsequent studies have confirmed the link.

CASE STUDY Eurofound

The largest and most important survey of working conditions – Eurofound's series of surveys covering the countries of the EU[4] – found in its most recent survey of workers that 24% of people working below 48 hours a week said work affected their health negatively and 22% believed it put their health and safety at risk. For those working 48 or more hours a week, however, the percentages increased to 35% and 31% respectively.

Aside from health conditions, excessive hours of working can manifest in changes in how you behave and feel, for example: tiredness and sleep problems; alcohol, smoking and drug misuse; reduced productivity; and irritability. Detailed advice on what to do is provided in our chapters on stress, mental health and musculoskeletal disorders. You should, in short, look to reduce your hours and adopt a healthier lifestyle through a balanced diet and regular exercise. Use your work rest breaks and holidays. And, given the correlation with strokes, you should have your doctor check your blood pressure regularly.

Your working time entitlements

Unusually for health and safety law, the legislation on working time is remarkably prescriptive in setting out your rights and entitlements. For most workers, the Working Time Regulations 1998[5] establish entitlements to a maximum working week, rest periods, night work restrictions and paid annual leave. If you are under the age of 18, the Regulations afford you extra protection (see chapter 14). If you are a lorry or coach driver, you are likely to be subject to different and complicated sets of rules, which we will outline later. There are also different rules for aircrew and seafarers. When reading about your rights, you should bear in mind that collective agreements between a union and employer can vary or exclude some of the provisions on daily, weekly and rest breaks and on night work.

Maximum working week

Under the Working Time Regulations 1998, you should work no more than 48 hours in a seven-day period (including overtime). This is usually averaged over 17 weeks, although it can be extended to 52 weeks by a collective agreement with a union or a workforce agreement with elected employee representatives. If your organization has 20 or fewer employees, the agreement must be with the individual employees. You can agree with your employer to work longer, either indefinitely or for a specified period, although you cannot opt out of the maximum working week if you work:[6]

- at night;
- on a ship, boat or plane;

- in the road transport industry, for example most delivery drivers;

- as an operator of vehicles covered by EU rules on drivers' hours, for example bus conductors; or

- as a security guard on a vehicle carrying high-value goods.

You may have to work more than 48 hours a week on average if you are in a job:[7]

- where 24-hour staffing is required;

- in the armed forces, emergency services or police;

- in security and surveillance;

- as a domestic servant in a private household;

- as a seafarer, in sea fishing or on vessels on inland waterways; or

- where working time is not measured and you are in control, for example a managing executive with control over your decisions.

The government provides advice on what counts towards the working week (for example, job-related training, paid overtime, time on call at the workplace, and travel between home and work if you do not have a fixed place of work); and what does not count (on-call time away from the workplace, paid or unpaid holiday and travel between home and a fixed place of work).[8] The TUC has produced a leaflet for people who have opted out of the maximum working week and who might want to opt back in.[9]

Work patterns and rest breaks

You are entitled to adequate rest breaks where the organization of your work puts your health and safety at risk. This arises particularly where the work is monotonous or the work-rate is predetermined. Notwithstanding this, you are entitled to a daily rest break, a daily rest period and a weekly rest period.

If you are working for more than six hours, you have a right to a 20-minute daily rest break away from your workstation. You should take this break during the day and not at the beginning or end. It can be a lunch break or tea break. Unless your contract of employment states otherwise, the break does not have to be paid and you do not have the right to smoking breaks.

You are also entitled to a daily rest period of 11 consecutive hours in any 24-hour period, and a further weekly rest period of 24 hours (consecutive where possible) in any seven-day period. Over a fortnight, this can be two 24-hour periods or a single 48-hour period.

The entitlements to rest periods do not apply in certain circumstances, including where: the activities involve a need for continuity of service or production; there are foreseeable busy periods; your workplace is a long way from home (for example an oil rig); or a shift worker changes shifts. In such circumstances, you are entitled to take the same amount of time as a 'compensatory break'.[10]

You will not be entitled to the three types of rest breaks if you work in:

- the armed forces, emergency services or police and are dealing with an exceptional situation;

- a job where you can choose what hours you work (for example a managing director) or where the hours are not measured; or

- sea, air or road transport, where you are generally covered by separate rules (see below).

Annual leave

You are entitled to 28 days' paid annual leave each year (which may include bank holidays). Those who work less than five days a week (or less than a full year) have pro rata entitlement. You must take the leave in the year in which it is due, unless prevented by sickness or by maternity or other statutory leave entitlement. You cannot receive a payment in lieu of the leave unless your employment is terminated. Your employer can require you to take leave on certain days and not to take leave on others, subject to giving you notice, the periods of which are specified in the Regulations.

Night work

We cover night work in detail in the next chapter. In short, night work occurs between 11pm to 6am unless an agreement is reached with your employer, in which case it must cover a seven-hour period that includes the hours between midnight and 5am. You are a night worker if at least three hours of your daily work are night work. As a night worker, you must not work for more than an average of eight hours in any 24-hour period over a 17-week period. If, however, you are a night worker and your job involves special hazards or heavy physical or mental strain, the limit is an absolute, ie there is no averaging.

Before you start night work, you are entitled to have a free health assessment and thereafter at regular intervals. Should a doctor inform your employer that you are suffering a health problem connected with your night work, your employer should transfer you, if possible, to non-night work that is suitable to you.

Securing your rights

Unfortunately, the Regulations are weakly enforced: there are few enforcement notices and fewer prosecutions. The HSE and local authorities enforce the maximum 48-hour week, night work limits and health assessments in the sectors for which they are responsible, while other regulators are responsible in certain sectors (see box).

You must complain to the Employment Tribunal if you are having problems with your rights under daily, weekly and rest breaks and annual leave (see chapter 19 on 'realizing your rights'). You must complain within three months and, if you are successful, you will receive compensation.

You must not suffer any detriment if you refuse to comply with a requirement made by your employer that contradicts your entitlements under the Regulations, or if you complain to your employer about its failure to grant you the rights. If you are dismissed as a result, the dismissal is unfair. You can get help on these issues from Acas (the Arbitration, Conciliation and Advisory Service).

Useful contacts

Acas Helpline Online: this is an automated helpline that covers many workplace issues: www.acas.org.uk/index. aspx?articleid=4489

Acas Helpline tel: 0300 123 1100

Air cabin crew – Civil Aviation Authority: www.caa.co.uk/home

HGV and PSV drivers – Driver and Vehicle Standards Agency: www.gov.uk/government/organisations/driver-and-vehicle-standards-agency

Seafarers and inland waterways workers – Maritime and Coastguard Agency: www.gov.uk/government/organisations/maritime-and-coastguard-agency

Nuclear installations workers – Office for Nuclear Regulation: www.onr.org.uk

Rail workers – Office of Rail and Road: orr.gov.uk

Drivers' hours

If you drive a goods vehicle or passenger-carrying vehicle, there are three sets of rules that might apply to your work, depending on the type of vehicle and the country in which you are driving. These are: EU rules; the European Agreement Concerning the Work of Crews of Vehicles Engaged in International Road Transport, which covers European countries not in the EU (but are now essentially the same as those of the EU and so not detailed here); and domestic rules. In addition, the Road Transport (Working Time) Regulations 2005 will apply to many drivers. As we noted at the start, the rules are detailed and complicated and we can here only give an overview.[11] Vehicles used in an emergency or for rescue operations are excluded from EU and domestic rules.

EU driving time rules

EU rules apply if the maximum permissible weight of your vehicle or vehicle combination is greater than 3.5 tonnes and you are driving in the EU (including the UK at the time of writing), a European Economic Area (EEA) country or Switzerland. The main EU rules, which are monitored by a tachograph, are that you must not drive for more than:

- nine hours in a day (although this can stretch to 10 hours twice a week);
- 56 hours in a week; and
- 90 hours in any two consecutive weeks.

You must also take:

- at least 11 hours of rest a day (you can reduce this to nine hours on three occasions between any two weekly rest periods);

- an unbroken rest period of 45 hours every week (you can reduce this to 24 hours every other week); and

- a break or breaks totalling at least 45 minutes after no more than four and a half hours' driving.

Domestic rules

You are covered by domestic rules if your vehicle weighs below 3.5 tonnes or is on a list of vehicles and uses that are exempted from the EU rules.[12] These include vehicles that: are incapable of moving at a speed higher than 40mph; have a maximum permissible mass of 7.5 tonnes and are used for the non-commercial transport of goods (for example, a charity lorry); have a maximum permissible mass of 7.5 tonnes and are used for carrying materials and equipment that the drivers use in the course of their work, do not go beyond a 100 km radius of the undertaking and where driving does not constitute the driver's main activity (for example, electricians or builders). Domestic rules do not apply if you drive for less than four hours in a day.

The domestic rules[13] limit driving a goods vehicle to a maximum of 10 hours, with no more than 11 hours on duty. Among other limitations are that if you are driving a passenger vehicle, you must take a rest break of at least 30 minutes after five hours and 30 minutes of driving, or, 45 minutes within any period of eight hours and 30 minutes. You must not work more than 16 hours between the times of starting and finishing work – including non-driving work and any times when you're off. You must take a rest of 10 hours before the first duty and immediately after the last duty in a working week.

And finally ...

If you operate a vehicle covered by the EU rules, you will also be subject to the Road Transport (Working Time) Regulations 2005[14] unless you are an occasional mobile worker (ie, if you work 10 or fewer days under the EU rules in a 26-week period, or 15 days over a longer period). Under the Regulations:

- your weekly working time must not exceed an average of 48 hours per week (normally over 17 weeks), although you can work up to a maximum of 60 hours in any single week. There is no opt-out;

- if you perform night work (between midnight and 4am for goods vehicles and between 1am and 5am for passenger vehicles), your working time must not exceed 10 hours in any 24-hour period, unless it is permitted under a collective or workforce agreement;

- you must not work more than six consecutive hours without taking a break;

- if your working hours total between six and nine hours, working time should be interrupted by a break or breaks (of at least 15 minutes) totalling at least 30 minutes, and at least 45 minutes if working beyond nine hours

- you are also covered by the requirements of the 1998 Regulations relating to paid annual leave and health checks for night workers.

If you drive a vehicle subject to the domestic rules or are an occasional mobile worker, you are affected by four provisions under the 1998 Regulations relating to: the 48-hour average maximum working week, although individuals can opt out; paid annual leave; health checks for night workers; and an entitlement to adequate rest.

Notes

1 Kivimäki P, Jokela M, Nyberg ST, et al. Long working hours and risk of coronary heart disease and stroke: a systematic review and meta-analysis of published and unpublished data for 603,838 individuals. *The Lancet.* 19 August 2015, vol. 386, 31 October 2015, www.thelancet.com/pdfs/journals/lancet/PIIS0140-6736(15)60295-1.pdf. A summary and analysis is available at: www.nhs.uk/news/neurology/working-long-hours-increases-stroke-risk

2 Institute for Employment Studies (2003) *Working long hours: a review of the evidence*, DTI, Employment Relations Research Series no.16, www.employment-studies.co.uk/system/files/resources/files/errs16_main.pdf

3 Health and Safety Laboratory (2003) *Working long hours*, HSL/2003/02, www.hse.gov.uk/research/hsl_pdf/2003/hsl03-02.pdf

4 Eurofound (2017) *Sixth European Working Conditions Survey. 2017 update*, www.eurofound.europa.eu/sites/default/files/ef_publication/field_ef_document/ef1634en.pdf

5 The Working Time Regulations 1998, SI 1998 No.1833, www.legislation.gov.uk/uksi/1998/1833/made/data.pdf

6 www.gov.uk/maximum-weekly-working-hours/weekly-maximum-working-hours-and-opting-out

7 www.gov.uk/maximum-weekly-working-hours

8 www.gov.uk/maximum-weekly-working-hours/calculating-your-working-hours

9 TUC, *Time's up for long hours*, www.tuc.org.uk/sites/default/files/tuc/optout.pdf

10 www.gov.uk/rest-breaks-work/compensatory-rest

11 Government advice on rules for driving hours is at: www.gov.uk/drivers-hours/eu-rules. The House of Commons Library produces briefing papers on the various rules governing driving hours, including Keter V and Smith L (2009), *Working time*

Directive and road transport, SN/BT/1758, researchbriefings.files.
parliament.uk/documents/SN01758/SN01758.pdf

12 A full list of vehicles and uses that are exempted from EU driving
hour rules is at: www.gov.uk/guidance/drivers-hours-goods-
vehicles/1-eu-and-aetr-rules-on-drivers-hours#exemptions-and-
derogations

13 www.gov.uk/drivers-hours/gb-domestic-rules

14 Road Transport (Working Time) Regulations 2005, SI 2005
No.639. www.legislation.gov.uk/uksi/2005/639/pdfs/
uksi_20050639_en.pdf

Chapter 10
Night and shift work

Millions of people in the UK work shifts, and the 24/7 society means that number is rising. But working when we should be sleeping takes its toll on our bodies as well as our social lives. Understanding more about our body clock can help reduce the health and safety risks associated with shift work.

The 24/7 society

Some 3.6 million people in the UK – that's 14% of the working population – do shift work most of the time.[1] More than 3.1 million people – or one in eight of all employees – in the UK work night shifts. Across the UK, that number is rising. Between 2011 and 2016, the number of people working shifts increased by 275,000.[2]

It's easy to forget how rapidly working patterns have changed. Before electric lighting was invented around 150 years ago, our working lives were regulated by sunrise and sunset.

Circadian rhythms and body clocks

Circadian rhythms are physical, mental and behavioural changes that follow a daily cycle. These rhythms – such as being awake during the day and sleeping at night – are driven by an internal body clock.

Circadian rhythms are found in practically every organism on the planet. Since life on Earth evolved 3.8 billion years ago, organisms have been exposed to trillions of dawns and dusks. This alternating cycle of day and night causes profound yet predictable changes in the environment, from how hot or cold it is to how much food is around. As a result, almost all organisms – from blue-green algae to humans – have evolved a body clock.

Body clocks are really important. They help plants and animals anticipate when day and night will come, allowing them to be prepared for the things that happen during the day and at night. Light is the main signal that resets the body clock to the 24-hour light–dark cycle created by the Earth's rotation.

Scientists first observed circadian rhythms in humans and other species hundreds of years ago, but they have been able to study them in detail only since the 1960s (see box). Developing better ways of growing cells in test tubes and decoding the genome of various species has allowed researchers to discover more about the mechanisms driving the body clock. This fundamental science has important real-world implications for millions of shift workers because it helps us understand how shift work disrupts our biology – and what we might do to minimize the disruption.

But to understand how disrupting our circadian rhythm threatens our wellbeing, we need to look at how these rhythms affect our physiology, metabolism and behaviour.

Clock research: a short history

It's only relatively recently that scientists have been begun to explore the body clock's mechanism, but people have been aware of circadian rhythms for hundreds of years. In 4th century BC Greece, Androsthenes described the daily movements of tamarind leaves and Hippocrates noted 24-hour patterns in human fevers. But it was a French astronomer, Jacques d'Ortous de Mairan, who in 1729 provided the first convincing evidence for a biological clock.

De Mairan was fascinated by mimosa, a tree which opens its leaves during the day and tucks them up at night. To find out more, he put the plants into 24-hour darkness. He found that even without light, the plants continued to open and close their leaves like clockwork. It was as if they could sense the sun despite its absence.

As recently as the 1950s, some scientists still disputed the idea of an internal body clock. During the 1960s, improvements in tissue culture allowed researchers to start studying the body clock in test tubes. In the 1970s, they discovered the pathway between the retina in the eye and the part of the brain that houses the clock. Finally, they found the clock itself – a small bunch of a few thousand cells in the hypothalamus. This they named the suprachiasmatic nucleus, or SCN.

Finding this master clock meant that scientists could begin to manipulate it experimentally, but it was only the discovery of the first clock genes, in the early 2000s, that at last allowed researchers to study how the clock actually works, and the how the SCN or master clock is wired up to the peripheral clocks that exist in all our other cells.

Health and the body clock

Being awake during the day and asleep at night is the most obvious outward sign of circadian rhythms. And although we are less aware of them, many other things inside our body follow a similar tempo. Our metabolism, our physiology and even the way our brains work run with a roughly 24-hour rhythm, and what our bodies do well during the day is very different from what happens at night.

Because we can't eat while we're asleep, during the day our liver, pancreas and gut are geared up to process food. During the day we produce more saliva, the rate at which our stomach empties is faster, our colon pulses more, and we burn glucose faster. These things don't happen by chance – they are driven by the body clock.

But it's not only our liver, pancreas and intestine that are affected. Levels of the stress hormone cortisol begin to rise before dawn. This ensures that by the time we wake up, we're ready to seize the day. Cortisol has major effects on our physiology – from blood pressure and cardiovascular system to metabolic rate and skeletal muscle – and affects our mood, concentration and creativity.

At dusk, while we prepare to withdraw from the world, these processes are turned down. Sleep, however, is more than mere absence of consciousness. At night, while we sleep, our body clock turns on systems that detoxify poisons, fight infection and promote growth, as well as processing information and consolidating memories.

All these things have an impact on our performance, so it's not surprising that many studies show a circadian variation in performance. In the 1890s, an American research student called Fletcher Dresslar spent six weeks timing himself tapping out Morse code every two hours from 8am to 6pm. It sounds tedious, but he discovered that his tapping speed varied. It speeded up from 8am to noon, slowed down after lunch, and then accelerated again so that by 6pm he could tap out messages faster than he did first thing in the morning.[3]

Swimmers can sprint faster over 50m – and tennis players serve more accurately – in the evening compared with the morning. Toothache is least painful in the morning, proofreading is more accurately done in the evening. More heart attacks – and more natural births – occur in the morning. All these things and more, from your bowel movements, sex drive and body temperature to glucose tolerance, and levels of the hunger and satiety hormones ghrelin and leptin all run like clockwork.[4] And all these examples suggest that being awake and at work when we should be asleep might have important results.

Shift work and the law

There's no legal definition of shift work, but it usually means work scheduled outside standard daytime hours or a work pattern that involves one employee replacing another on the same job during a 24-hour period.

It's your employer's legal responsibility to ensure their employees' health and safety; this includes organizing shift work so that risks associated with fatigue are removed, controlled or removed.

Your employer also has general duties under the Health and Safety at Work etc Act 1974 and the Management of Health and Safety at Work Regulations 1999 to manage the risks associated with shift work.

Your employer also has a legal duty to consult employees about health and safety matters and take your views into account before reaching any decision. This is covered by the Safety Representatives and Safety Committees Regulations and the Health and Safety (Consultation with Employees) Regulations 1996.

The Working Time Regulations 1998 cover minimum legal requirements on working time, and make some specific provisions for night workers, including a limit of an average of 8 hours work in each 24-hour period; a right to 11 hours consecutive rest a day, a day off each week, a rest break if the working day is longer than 6 hours; and a right to free health assessments.[5]

Shift work and health

Not surprisingly, many scientific studies have found that being awake when our body clock thinks we should be asleep has far-reaching consequences for health and safety, and accidents are merely the most immediate risk.

Some of the world's worst industrial disasters, from Chernobyl and Three Mile Island to Bhopal and the Exxon Valdez, occurred at night and many researchers say that's not a coincidence. Other statistics suggest the same: drowsiness causes some 20% of traffic accidents on major roads, and losing even one hour's sleep when clocks change to British Summer Time results in 20% more traffic accidents. Being awake for 24 hours, says chronobiologist Professor Russel Foster of the University of Oxford, impairs performance to the same degree as being over the drink driving limit.[6]

Evidence also suggests that shift work increases the risk of many serious health conditions. Nurses are among the best studied shift workers, and research shows that night shifts are associated with increased incidence of type 2 diabetes, gastrointestinal disorders, heart disease, obesity, depression, memory problems, breast cancer and colorectal cancer.

Sleep disruption also affects our emotions and mental health. Recent research by Foster's colleague Professor Daniel Freeman found that treating insomnia with cognitive behavioural therapy could reduce mental health problems such as anxiety, depression and paranoia. Even our resistance to infection is not immune to the impact of sleep loss. Having a flu jab is much less effective – resulting in 50% fewer antibodies – after four hours' sleep rather than eight hours.

As well as biological effects, shift work can also have an impact on your work-life balance, and in particular on your home life and relationships.[7] Living against our natural rhythms is clearly associated with range of health risks. So, is there anything you and your employer can do to reduce those risks?

Healthier shift work

For all of these reasons, it would be fair to say that there is no such thing as healthy shift work. However, it is definitely possible to make it less unhealthy. Even though we don't fully understand the complex mechanisms at work, experts believe that we know enough to try to mitigate the health issues associated with shift work.

One of the more recent and most interesting is the idea of chronotype. While we all have an internal clock, some of us have a distinct preference for getting up and going to bed early, while others prefer to get up and go to sleep later. A German chronobiologist, Professor Till Roenneberg, developed a quiz called the Munich ChronoType Questionnaire to study these so-called chronotypes. Since 2000, thousands of people have done the questionnaire, revealing that about 10–15% of us are larks or morning types and 10–15% of us are owls or evening types, with most of us somewhere in between. If you want to find out more about your chronotype, you can do the questionnaire online (see box).

Munich sleep questionnaire

Some people describe themselves as larks or night owls. This is down to a mixture of factors from genetics to age and gender. Scientists call this your 'chronotype' and they have developed a simple questionnaire that lets you find out more about your chronotype.

Developed at Ludwig-Maximilian University in Munich by Professor Till Roenneberg and his team, the Munich ChronoType Questionnaire asks you to record your bedtime and what time you wake up on work days and free days (the latter without an alarm clock) over four weeks.

Knowing your chronotype can help you work out which kind of shifts might suit you better. You can find out more about the Munich ChronoType Questionnaire online.[8]

Your chronotype is the result of several factors including age, gender and genetics, and varies throughout our lives. Sleep habits change markedly with age, with teenagers being much more owlish and older people more likely to be up with the larks. And your chronotype will also affect your ability to cope with different shifts. If you're an owl, being forced to do morning shifts will be much harder than doing late shifts, for example.

The key message is that as far as shift work's concerned, there is no one-size-fits-all solution, so we need to be more aware of chronotypes. According to Professor Russell Foster of the University of Oxford: 'People ask what's the best shift schedule? The answer is that there isn't one, because it depends on whether you're a morning or evening type. One type does not fit all, so chronotype is critically important.'[9]

Appropriate nutrition is also crucial. Settling into a healthy diet is relatively easy to do, and of course will also have a major positive impact on your health. We know that our digestive system isn't optimized to process food at night, and that night shifts are associated with more obesity and cardiovascular disease, so it's worth paying attention to what – and when – you eat if you're working shifts.

We've seen that missing sleep messes with our bodies' hunger hormones, resulting in higher levels of the hunger hormone ghrelin and lower levels of leptin, the hormone that controls how satiated you feel. That's why, if you're tired, you will crave high sugar, high fat foods. The TUC says that employers should make sure that night workers have access to the same facilities as day workers, including hot meals, drinks and rest areas.[10] If you take your own food into work, think about packing small portions of high protein, low fat, low sugar meals that are easier to digest. The National Sleep Foundation has lots of tips for shift workers, including advice on what foods to eat.[11]

As a society, we also need to radically rethink our attitudes to sleep. According to Professor Matthew Walker, director of the

Center for Human Sleep Science at the University of California, Berkeley, we are in the middle of a global sleep loss epidemic. Sleep has an image problem, he says, because we stigmatize sleep and think it's lazy and slothful. But Walker and other sleep researchers warn that we ignore sleep at our peril. Sleep is not a luxury, sleep deprivation is not a badge of honour, and public health bodies should be stressing the importance of sleep with the same vigour as they promote health messages about diet, smoking, alcohol and exercise.[12]

In the USA, for example, the National Sleep Foundation recommends how much sleep people should get depending on their age. The recommendations, which are based on a thorough review of the scientific evidence, say that teenagers should get 8–10 hours sleep per night, adults between 18 and 64 years old should get 7–9 hours and for older adults (65+) it's best to get 7–8 hours' sleep.[13]

In 2018, Business in the Community and Public Health England produced the first ever sleep and recovery toolkit for UK employers. It offers information and advice on what it describes as 'the increasingly damaging sleep-loss epidemic affecting the nation'.[14]

There are many other things your employer should be doing to reduce the health risks associated with shift work. As well as how they operate their shift schedules (see box), employers should ensure that shift workers have access to more frequent health screening. We know that sleep-wake disruption is associated with loss of vigilance, impulsivity and memory loss, as well as cardiovascular disease, type 2 diabetes and metabolic syndrome, so screening could help identify these problems before they become pathological. If your employer does not provide such access, you should speak to your trade union rep or the occupational health service where you work.

What can I do to improve my health and wellbeing?

If you work shifts, there are many things you can do to improve your health and wellbeing. Several organizations, including the HSE, the Sleep Council and the National Sleep Federation, provide plenty of practical advice that's available free on the web.

When you work shifts, driving to and from work can be risky. Think about whether you could take a taxi, use public transport or share driving. If that's not possible, then drive carefully and stop if you feel sleepy.

Getting enough good quality sleep is essential for health and wellbeing, and sleep loss and fatigue can be significant problems for shift workers. People often don't sleep as well during the day, so it's important to make sure that your bedroom is completely dark, cool and quiet. Use blackout blinds or curtains, turn off your telephone and try using earplugs.

Being relaxed before you go to bed can help you sleep better. This might mean reading a book or having a warm bath. And avoid vigorous exercise, alcohol, caffeine and other stimulants for several hours before you go to bed.

We've seen how circadian rhythm disruption affects your appetite, your digestive system and your metabolism so eating a healthy diet is really important if you work shifts. Eat fruit and vegetables rather than foods that are high in fat and sugar. Try eating smaller, lighter meals rather than one large meal. You can also try preparing meals before your shift so that you have something healthy to hand, and remember to drink enough fluids. Your employer should provide you with access to the same hot food and drinks facilities as day workers, but if there's only a vending machine full of crisps and chocolate then speak to your trade union representative.

Try to avoid relying on stimulants (such as caffeine and cigarettes) and sedatives. Instead, try taking moderate exercise before your shift, keep the light bright and take regular, short breaks to help you stay alert. And remember that regular exercise will improve your health and your sleep.

Many apps have been developed to help people sleep. Sleepful.me, for example, is a self-help programme that has been developed through a series of publicly-funded research studies and clinical trials in the UK.[15]

What should my employer be doing?

Changing your own habits can help reduce the health risks associated with working shifts, but there is much that your employer can – and should – be doing. The TUC recommends that employers and trade unions should ensure that night-working is only introduced where necessary, and when it is introduced, existing workers should not be forced to work nights.

Shift patterns should be negotiated between trade unions and employers, and workers should have some control over their rotas so that the shifts they work are best suited to their individual circumstances. Self-rostering and being able to switch shifts can also help. Workers should always have sufficient notice of their shift patterns so they can make arrangements well in advance, making changes at short notice should be avoided, and remuneration paid to people working nights should properly reflect the likely additional costs of childcare and inconvenience that night shifts can entail.[16]

Permanent night shifts should be replaced with rotating shifts if possible. Research by the HSE suggests that rotating shifts every two to three days is best or, failing that, slow rotations of at least three weeks. Weekly or fortnightly rotations are least comfortable for workers, whose bodies will just have started to adapt to the new pattern when it is switched again. Forward-rotating schedules (moving from morning to afternoon to night shifts) are better than backward-rotating ones in terms of sleep loss and fatigue.[17]

The HSE's guidance on shift work provides information on different shift patterns, advice for employers on assessing and managing the risks of shift work, and practical advice for shift workers on how to improve health and wellbeing.[18]

Notes

1   HSE (2006) *Managing Shiftwork*. www.hse.gov.uk/pUbns/priced/hsg256.pdf

2   TUC (2015) *A hard day's night*. www.tuc.org.uk/sites/default/files/AHardDaysNight.pdf

3   Foster R and Kreitzman L (2017) *Circadian Rhythms: A very short introduction*, Oxford University Press

4   Foster, Kreitzman. *Circadian Rhythms*

5   HSE (2006) *Managing Shiftwork*

6   Lockley SW and Foster R (2012). *Sleep: A very short introduction*, Oxford University Press

7   TUC. *A hard day's night*

8   www.thewep.org/documentations/mctq

9   Allen B (2017) 'Clocking on', *IOSH Magazine*, December

10 TUC. *A hard day's night*

11 National Sleep Foundation: https://sleepfoundation.org/shift-work/content/tips-healthy-eating-and-exercising-when-working-shifts

12 Walker M (2018) *Why We Sleep*, Scribner, New York

13 National Sleep Foundation (2015) *National Sleep Foundation recommends new sleep times*. https://sleepfoundation.org/press-release/national-sleep-foundation-recommends-new-sleep-times

14 BITC (2018). *Sleep and recovery: A toolkit for employers.*
https://wellbeing.bitc.org.uk/sites/default/files/bitc_phe_sleep_
recovery_toolkit-final-18.01.18.pdf

15 Sleepful: https://sleepful.me

16 TUC. *A hard day's night*

17 Acas: www.acas.org.uk/index.aspx?articleid=3877

18 HSE. *Managing Shiftwork*

Chapter 11
Physical wellbeing and health initiatives

What we eat, how active we are and our smoking and drinking habits all have a massive impact on our long-term health. Obesity is linked to increased risk of diabetes, heart disease and some cancers. Being physically active is important for heart health and weight management. Eating enough fruit and vegetables reduces the risk of heart disease, stroke and some cancers.

Because of this, the government publishes guidelines on exercise, diet and alcohol consumption. The guidelines[1] recommend:

- Taking 150 minutes of moderate exercise, or 75 minutes' vigorous exercise, each week.
- Doing muscle strengthening activity like yoga or carrying heavy shopping at least two days a week.
- Minimizing how much time we spend sitting down for extended periods.
- Quitting smoking.
- Drinking less than 14 units of alcohol a week.
- Eating at least five portions of a variety of fruit and veg a day.

According to the annual *Healthj Survey for England*, 26% of adults are obese; only 66% of men and 58% of women take enough exercise; 20% of men and 16% of women smoke; 24% of men and 28% of women eat five portions of fruit and veg a day.

Our work has a major impact on our health, and work that's unsafe or unhealthy has a negative impact on our physical and mental health. Physical and mental health are also closely connected and many studies, including Mind's Get Set to Go campaign, show that being more physically active is good for our mental health (see chapter 1).[2]

The workplace is an important setting for encouraging healthier lifestyles. We spend a significant proportion of our time at work, so employers have a major role to play in helping us to eat more healthily, be more physically active, and address unhealthy behaviours such as smoking.[3]

Successful wellbeing and health initiatives depend on as many workers as possible taking part, so involving staff and trade unions at the outset is vital. It's also good practice to collect baseline data via an employee needs assessment so that initiatives can be evaluated and shared.[4]

The following case studies illustrate a range of wellbeing and health initiatives that should be easy to replicate in your workplace. They cover a range of activities, from healthy eating to physical activity, different sizes of organization in different sectors, plus local authorities and trade unions which offer workplace wellbeing programmes. If you're inspired by any of the ideas, speak to your trade union representative, occupational health service, HR department or manager.

CASE STUDY   Living Streets – walking local, everyday journeys

As a nation, we are walking a third less today than we did 20 years ago. Within just a couple of generations, we've effectively engineered walking out of our lives. That matters, because walking is good for our physical and mental health. Regular physical activity reduces your risk of dementia by up to 30%, heart disease by 35%, type 2 diabetes by 40%, depression by 30% and colon cancer by 30%. These are such huge benefits that if physical activity was a drug, it would be classed as a wonder drug.

The UK Chief Medical Officers recommend that adults should aim to do at least 150 minutes of moderate intensity physical activity each week in bouts of 10 minutes or more. As well as being physically active, we also need to spend less time sitting down for long periods. Walking is one of the simplest ways to build this activity into your week and there are lots of ways that your workplace can help to make it a habit.

Living Streets is the UK charity for everyday walking. Set up in 1929, its early campaigns led to the UK's first zebra crossings. Today, Living Streets is working with government, schools and workplaces to get more people back on their feet. 'We want to create a nation where walking is the natural choice for local, everyday journeys,' the charity says.

Because walking can play a key role in promoting wellbeing at work, Living Streets has produced a range of information and initiatives for workplaces. Walking Works is a 16-page booklet full of tips to encourage staff to build walking into their working day from how to organize walking meetings or set up a 'food exclusion zone' to tempt people further from their desks to building more walking into your commute to work, and #Try20 is Living Streets' top tips to get 20 minutes more walking into your day.

Living Streets also offers a range of bespoke consultancy, project management and behaviour-change initiatives. In 2017, the Phoenix Group asked the charity to help get its staff walking more. Living Streets developed a special self-guided walking trail using the online walking app Crumbs. The trail was launched during National Walking Month in May with a lunchtime led-walk, and guides walkers on a 1.4-mile trail around the City of London, taking in secret gardens and historic places at the same time as clocking up 3,036 steps and burning 140 calories. At Phoenix's offices at Wythall, Birmingham, Living Streets created a walk within the site's 42 acres, taking in various points of natural interest, including a wildflower bank, bee box, insect hotel and Koi Mirror Carp.

In Stoke-on-Trent, Living Streets combined a walking initiative with corporate social responsibility (CSR). Staff at Michelin joined forces with the Canal and River Trust to spruce up a section of the Cauldon Canal. By clearing vegetation and painting signs and monuments, they created a safer, more accessible route that the whole community can use to walk to work and during working hours.

You can find out more about these initiatives at:

Living Streets www.livingstreets.org.uk

Public Health England (2016) Health matters: Getting every adult active every day. www.gov.uk/government/publications/health-matters-getting-every-adult-active-every-day/health-matters-getting-every-adult-active-every-day

Public Health England (2016) Health matters: There's never been a better time to promote active travel. https://publichealthmatters.blog.gov.uk/2016/08/30/health-matters-theres-never-been-a-better-time-to-promote-active-travel

CASE STUDY North East Better Health at Work
Award – Busy Bees

Award schemes can be a great way to begin – and sustain – a health at work programme. They provide advice, information and support to help you design activities that will suit your workplace, and recognition to reward what your workplace achieves.

The North East Better Health at Work Award (BHAWA)[5] is a free, flexible scheme that's open to all employers in the North East and Cumbria. Run by the Northern TUC in partnership with local councils and the NHS, there are four levels of award from bronze, silver, gold and continuing excellence, plus a special ambassador award.

Each award involves meeting certain criteria and for the higher-level awards, these extend beyond individual workplaces to promote health in local communities and among the families of staff. Each employer needs to have at least two health advocates among their workforce. Health advocates are key to the scheme's success, so they need full support from management, and time to deliver and develop a health action plan with the support of a Workplace Health Improvement Specialist from BHAWA.

So far, more than 400 employers in the region have taken part in the awards. Their staff benefit from greater access to health information and interventions. At the same time, employers benefit from happier, healthier workers who are more productive and take fewer days off sick.

Busy Bees Newcastle[6] has been part of BHAWA since 2011. Part of a national chain of nurseries, Busy Bees Newcastle has 40 staff and cares for 200 children; its manager, Victoria Solomon, decided to get involved in the awards after being approached by a BHAWA rep. Since then, Busy Bees Newcastle has achieved bronze, silver and gold and in 2018 won both the continuing excellence and ambassador awards. 'It's a really proud moment for us,' says Victoria. 'Our nursery is rated outstanding and we have really high standards, so anything we can do to maintain that and focus on staff as well as the children is great.'

What she likes best about BHAWA is the support and guidance that the scheme provides. 'The staff at Northumbria Healthcare are always there for you, providing lots of advice, ideas and contacts to help you run the activities. Our staff really value what we've achieved – they say they feel healthier and so do I.'

Victoria is one of two health advocates at Busy Bees Newcastle and together they've delivered a huge range of activities from healthy eating and healthy weight to exercise and mental health: 'We carry out a wellbeing questionnaire twice a year so that staff can tell us what they need from a health and wellbeing point of view, what they want to achieve and how we can support them.'

Some of the most memorable events employ an element of fun to communicate serious health messages. One event focussed on cancer awareness. 'We borrowed model testicles and breasts from the BHAWA team,' Victoria says. 'We set up the models – which contain lumps – in a private room at lunchtime. We did raise a smile, but we also got some really important information across and gave out leaflets that staff could take away and use or share with their families.'

CASE STUDY   Cornwall Council – helping to make small businesses healthier

Working for a small business shouldn't be a barrier to setting up a health and wellbeing programme at work, as Cornwall Council shows. Covering Cornwall and the Isles of Scilly, it's the largest non-metropolitan unitary authority in the country and it's unique because 98% of its businesses are small and medium-sized enterprises (SMEs).

Although the county has a few large employers (the Council itself has 5,000 staff and the NHS 3,000), every workplace – from local government, private sector and charities to SMEs and larger employers – can sign up to get free support and advice from the Cornwall and Isles of Scilly Healthy Workplace Programme.[7]

The programme is built around the Healthy Workplace Award, which provides a framework to encourage employers to think about ways of improving the health and wellbeing of staff. It consists of 10 topics – from specific issues such as sun safety and preventing back pain to business issues like leadership. 'A dual responsibility is needed,' says the Council, 'individuals can make healthy choices and the workplace can ensure the healthier choice is the easier choice.'

Once an employer has signed up to the programme, they'll be visited by one of the team and taken through everything that's on offer, including healthy weight sessions and mental health first aid training, and introduced to other local businesses which are part of the programme. 'We've linked up lots of small employers on industrial estates so they can meet up at lunch for health walks,' says Amy Bromfield, one of the Council's workplace health advisers.

Workplaces are supported with monthly newsletters, quarterly health training, a twice-yearly forum with speakers so that employers can take new ideas back to their workplaces, and the annual conference and awards ceremony. 'There's lots online for employers to access, so they can be as involved as they like,' she says.

The team also organizes the annual Beach Games and provides a range of on-site sessions, including a 12-week healthy weight and healthy eating course. It kicks off by measuring people's body composition so that everyone can take away a printout of their muscle mass, hydration and metabolic age. There's a workshop on healthy eating, including tips for packed lunches and night workers, as well as advice for on-site catering. People's progress is assessed when the team returns three months later and the results in many workplaces is 'amazing', says Amy.

So far, more than 400 workplaces have signed up and one of Cornwall's larger employers, the Environment Agency, joined the Healthy Workplace

Award scheme in 2016. Thanks to a big focus on healthy weight, including eat well workshops and advice on sugar and food labelling, plus a campaign to combat prolonged sitting by providing adjustable sit/stand desks and promoting standing meetings, there's been a 30% reduction in the number of staff with obesity and a doubling of the percentage of staff classed as at a 'healthy weight'.

CASE STUDY   Anglian Water – Random acts of wildness

There's an increasing amount of evidence to show that exposure to nature is good for us. Getting out more – to feed the birds, have a walk or get involved in some conservation volunteering – can help reduce high blood pressure and anxiety as well as boost mood and energy levels.

In 2016, the University of Derby measured the impact of the Wildlife Trusts' 30 Days Wild – its annual challenge to do one wild thing each day during June. The researchers found that after taking part in the challenge, the number of people who rated their health as 'excellent' increased by 30%. The Conservation Volunteers also run a Green Gym scheme to inspire people to improve their mental and physical health at the same time as helping the environment. A study of Green Gym volunteers in 2016 found that after volunteering for three months, people were doing 50% more exercise, eating more fresh fruit and veg, and 80% had lost weight.

Inspired by nature as well as by what works, Anglian Water decided to introduce an innovative idea into its workplace wellbeing programme. Called Biophilia, to reflect our natural affinity for the natural world, the summer 2017 campaign teamed up Anglian Water's occupational health and wellbeing team with its Potting Shed Club, which helps its customers to save water in the garden. To encourage the workforce to get out into nature, all 4,700 employees received a packet of seeds – including drought-loving species like oregano – and some tools about how to improve their mental health. 'We know walking's good for physical and mental health,' says Jonathan Hill, Anglian Water's Occupational Health Manager, 'but it empowers employees to create something new by sowing seeds, it's a form of mindfulness, therefore it can be seen as a mental health intervention.'

As part of Anglian Water's next campaign, which focuses on musculoskeletal disorders, bike desks will soon be arriving in each of the water company's three main sites. They'll be located in breakout spaces so that staff can pop down and cycle while they work. It's a bit of fun, but it might have longer-lasting benefits too.

'Using the bike desks, there'll be a cycle to Paris competition between the sites. We'll decorate the breakout areas with French flags and as well as encouraging team work, it might also encourage staff to get out more on their own bikes,' he says. 'We're all about a positive wellbeing culture and doing that means behaviour change – giving lots of little nudges and reminders about how important it is to stay active.'

You can find out more about these initiatives at:

30 Days Wild www.wildlifetrusts.org/30DaysWild

Green Gym www.tcv.org.uk/greengym/what-green-gym

POSTnote (2016) Green space and health. http://researchbriefings. parliament.uk/ResearchBriefing/Summary/POST-PN-0538?utm_ source=directory&utm_medium=website&utm_campaign=PN538

CASE STUDY　Public Health England – One You

If your workplace doesn't yet have a health and wellbeing programme, or you're self-employed and work by yourself, you can use free online tools and mobile apps to improve your health. In 2016, Public Health England launched One You, a new website and a series of free apps designed to help people in their 40s and 50s make simple changes that will improve their health.[8]

There's a 10-minute quiz that asks about your weight and your mood as well as your sleep and your stress levels. It encourages you to think about what you're eating and drinking and how active you are, and then uses the information you provide to offer concrete suggestions. And if you sign up, you'll get emailed regular tips and tricks to keep you motivated.

There's also a series of free apps, including the popular Couch to 5k running programme and the new Active 10 walking tracker. Just 10 minutes of brisk walking a day can improve your health and help you feel better. Developed in collaboration with the University of Sheffield, Sheffield Hallam University and the National Centre for Sport and Exercise Medicine, the Active 10 app shows you how many brisk 10-minute walks you're taking and how to fit more into your day.

Other resources

There are lots of resources online to help you look after your physical wellbeing and health. To get you started, a few are listed below:

BITC *Physical activity, healthy eating and healthier weight: a toolkit for employers.* https://wellbeing.bitc.org.uk/sites/ default/files/bitc_phe_physical_activity-healthy_ eating-healthier_weight_toolkit_final_updated_9_ march_ 2018.pdf

NHS Choices *Eating a balanced diet.* www.nhs.uk/Livewell/ Goodfood/Pages/Healthyeating.aspx

The *Change4Life Food Scanner* app lets you look up the sugar, saturated fat and salt in everyday foods and drinks by scanning the barcodes of more than 140,000 products. https://apps.beta.nhs.uk/change4life-food-scanner

NHS Physical activity guidelines for adults. www.nhs.uk/ Livewell/fitness/Pages/physical-activity-guidelines-for-adults. aspx

London Healthy Workplace Charter www.london.gov.uk/ what-we-do/health/healthy-workplace-charter

Natural England (2016) A review of nature-based interventions for mental health care. http://publications.naturalengland. org.uk/publication/4513819616346112

Notes

1 Public Health England (2016) *Health matters: getting every adult active every day*. www.gov.uk/government/publications/health-matters-getting-every-adult-active-every-day/health-matters-getting-every-adult-active-every-day

2 NCSEM Mind: Get Set to Go. www.ncsem.org.uk/impact/mind-get-set-to-go

3 NHS Digital (2016) *Health survey for England*. https://digital.nhs.uk/media/34551/Health-Survey-for-England-2016-Summary-of-key-findings/pdf/HSE2016-summary

4 TUC (2015) *Work and well-being: A trade union resource*. www.tuc.org.uk/sites/default/files/work-and-well-being-2015.pdf

5 North East Better Health at Work Award: www.betterhealthatworkne.org

6 Busy Bees Newcastle: www.busybeeschildcare.co.uk/nursery/newcastle

7 Cornwall and Isles of Scilly Workplace Health Award: www.behealthyatwork.org

8 One You: www.nhs.uk/oneyou

Chapter 12
Access to occupational health advice

At many points in this book, you will have come across our advice to consult your GP or your employer's occupational health service (OHS) if you believe you have a health problem that might be linked to your work. Your employer may also have an Employee Assistance Programme (EAP), which typically will give you access to a telephone or web-based advice line and counselling services. The reality, however, is that a majority of workers do not have access to an OHS or even an EAP, which means that the GP is most often your first port of call.

Visiting your GP

GPs are under significant time pressures and the average duration of an appointment does not always facilitate a full discussion of work-related factors that may be affecting your condition. It is important, therefore, that you make the most of your consultation time. Think carefully about the points in the box before you see your GP and then make sure you cover each point during your appointment. Your GP may refer you for treatment or issue a 'fit note' (see box).

Points to raise with your GP

The following covers the information that you should provide to your GP if you believe that your symptoms may be related to your job:

- the symptoms and duration of your condition (and whether any of your colleagues are suffering similar or unusual symptoms);
- whether your symptoms change when you are not at work;
- the type of work that you do;
- whether you work shifts or unusual patterns;
- any particular pressures, targets or constraints under which you work;
- whether you are exposed to any chemicals or potentially dangerous substances;
- your previous employment – some conditions, for example deafness and asbestos-related diseases, may have originated many years earlier; and
- whether there are any non-work factors that might be relevant, for example a hobby.

Your GP should, in any case, be increasingly aware of the need to consider an occupational role in your condition. The Society and Faculty of Occupational Medicine (SOM and FOM, which is the professional and educational body for occupational medicine (OM)) have been running a *Why occupational health?* campaign[1] since early 2017 to increase the understanding across all health professionals of the relationship between health and work. One of the campaign's aims is to encourage GPs and primary care teams to consider whether a job is making a patient ill and whether the health status of a patient is adversely affecting his or her capacity or fitness for work. The SOM has also produced a short guide on OH for workers and their representatives.[2] This emphasizes that OH nurses and doctors have a professional duty to protect your confidentiality and to inform you how your health information is recorded and used, and of your right of access to your personal information. They will not disclose any information without your consent, unless someone may be at risk of serious harm.

Should your employer's OHS – through surveillance, screening or testing – find a medical issue, it will likely want to inform your GP. Again, this needs your written and informed consent. You should also make sure, wherever possible, that your GP supplies information to your OH department rather than line or personnel managers. Whereas your GP might advocate for you, an OH department will give impartial advice to you and your employer.

Fit notes

If you are off work for more than seven days, your doctor will issue a Statement of Fitness for Work. The government introduced the 'fit note', as it is commonly known, in 2010, replacing the 'sick note' in recognition of evidence that being out of work is bad for you and that the longer you are on sick leave the less likely it is you will return to work.

The main changes were that the note can now state that you 'may' be fit for work in general rather than are merely unfit for work. Importantly, your GP can give general advice about how your health issues may affect what you can do at work and suggest ways in which your employer might help you return to work through, for example a phased return, amended duties, reduced or altered hours, working from home, providing a mentor, changes to the work station or workplace and an occupational health assessment. These are suggestions, however, and not binding on your employer. The government has produced guidance for employers that you may find helpful.[3]

Analysis shows that GPs issued an average of one fit note for every 48 patients in England aged 18–65 years in 2016/17.[4] Of the notes, 6.5% classified the patient as 'may be fit for work', of which 80% recommended an adaptation in the workplace, working hours or duties. Of the fit notes, 31.3% with a known diagnosis were for mental and behavioural disorders, and 18% for diseases of the musculoskeletal system and connective tissue.

OH specialists

If you are referred to an occupational health specialist by your GP or your employer's OHS or under your employer's private medical scheme, you should check that the specialist is appropriately qualified. TUC guidance,[5] which is based on FOM advice, states that doctors should have one of the following sets of letters after their name: DOccMed, AFOM, MFOM or FFOM (see box). Without these letters, the TUC believes that is likely that the practitioners will have only what they call minimal training in OM, and not have 'the qualifications, experience and checks that will assure competency'. You can easily check the details of the physician on the GMC register.[6]

Check your doctor's acronym

- **DOccMed** (Diploma in Occupational Medicine). There are medical practitioners – often GPs – who have a special interest and training in occupational medicine (OM) but who are not specialists. They should nonetheless have the DOccMed, which the HSE recommends as the minimum standard for those working in OM. Diploma holders, advises the TUC, can 'give basic day to day advice and will have some understanding of the issues that affect health and work. They will be able to do health assessments etc, but would need to consult a specialist in many more complex situations';[7]

- **AFOM** (Associate Member of the Faculty of Occupational Medicine (FOM)), which demonstrates core knowledge in OM theory and practice. Associate membership offers a professional pathway for doctors who work in OM but are not in an approved training post; and

- **MFOM** and **FFOM** (Member and Fellow of the FOM), which mean the doctor will have will have completed the approved training in OM. A specialist doctor or consultant in OM must be listed on the GMC's specialist register and will usually be a MFOM or FFOM.

Referrals to other specialists (with different acronyms) will also be appropriate where other specialisms are needed, for example in chest medicine, dermatology and rheumatology. Referrals will also often be to a non-medical practitioner, such as a physiotherapist, nurse or podiatrist, who will be registered with their own professional bodies. The TUC emphasizes that they should not be seen as second best, although generally they can only assess and treat specific injury or illness, rather than diagnose.

Doctors on the GMC medical register can also act as an expert for your employer or your employer's insurer, but this does not mean that they have had any specialist training. They may, according to the TUC, have 'only limited knowledge' of many of the areas that they should be dealing with, although it does not mean that they are incapable of dealing with some issues.

Occupational health services

You may be fortunate and work for an employer that has access to a multidisciplinary occupational health services (OHS). This may be in-house or an external contracted provider. In-house OHSs will vary in numbers and types of staffing, but will comprise one or more of the following – a physician, hygienist, nurse or other specialist. Multi-disciplinary services will carry out various functions that may at some point help you, including:

- a post-offer health assessment or pre-employment examination;

- consultation if you are feeling unwell;

- assessments of your health and workplace if you are suffering from a problem that you believe may be linked to your work;

- early detection of any problems through health screening, surveillance and testing;

- early interventions, with an improved chance of speeding your recovery and reducing the amount of time for which you might be off work, for example physiotherapy (for which you might wait for a long time on the NHS);

- promotion of good health and wellbeing initiatives;

- immunizations and preventive medicines if you are exposed to infectious diseases at work or during foreign travel;

- a check of your medical capability to return to work after absence due to illness of injury; and

- advice on reasonable adjustments so that persons with health conditions and disabilities can remain in or return to work.

Checking out your OHS

If you are referred to an OHS or OH physiotherapist practice, you should check that it is SEQOHS-accredited (Safe, Effective, Quality Occupational Health Service). Your employer should have done this, but it is worth making sure. The SEQOHS is the only OH accreditation scheme that is recognized by the government, occupational doctors, the TUC and employers' organizations. The TUC, which offers a free guide to help you check your OH provider,[8] believes that accreditation under the voluntary scheme helps give a guarantee that the provider's OH staff are appropriately qualified and that the provider has been regularly audited against standards. At the time of writing, there were 207 accredited providers and another 178 working towards accreditation. They are listed alphabetically on the SEQOHS website, alongside details of their certification.[9] You should always check the downloadable certificate to make sure that it is accredited to the part of the standard that covers the service you will be receiving.

The problem of access

Government figures show that less than four in 10 employees (38%) in the UK have access to an OHS.[10] The chances of OHS access increase with organizational size, from 10% (1–50 employees) to 52% (500+ employees). Rates also vary between sectors, with a 2008 review by Dame Carol Black[11] noting that 1% of agriculture, forestry and fishing workers had access to occupational physicians compared with 43% of health and social services workers. A 2016 report from an all-party group of MPs[12] warned that the number of OHSs and occupational physicians in the UK is inadequate for the demand and that 'few' workers had access to OHS and 'even fewer' to a doctor who had a speciality in OM. The MPs concluded that the inequality of access in the UK to occupational physicians is 'unrivalled compared to any other northern European country' and that the UK needs three times its current number of occupational physicians.[13]

Unfortunately, the availability of such services looks set to reduce still further. Figures from the General Medical Council[14] show that the number of OM specialists fell by 5% between 2010 and 2013 alone, and the MPs noted that the number of trainees specializing in OM in 2015 was around a third the number in 2002. The problem is exacerbated by the fact that the percentage of doctors over the age of 50 is higher for OM (64%) than for any other specialism, which means a significant proportion of doctors will be retiring from the profession imminently. Aside from the loss of provision, it also means there will be fewer specialists to train the next generation. Health Education England boosted the intake of trainees in 2016/17 but the MPs point out that the number (46) is 'inadequate'.

At the same time, OHSs will have to cope with greater calls on their services, with increasing numbers of people with health conditions and disabilities able or expected to work providing their employer makes reasonable adjustments. Furthermore, the deferred pension age means that increasing numbers of people will have to work for longer (and are more likely to develop health problems with age).

Fit for Work service

All but 0.1% of UK's businesses are small employers and 60% of employees work in a SME. Size and economies mean that SMEs will not have internal OH advice and, at best, will use a contracted-out service. The growth in recent year of smaller enterprises, temporary and insecure work, zero-hours contracts and other new ways of working leaves more and more workers unlikely to have access to an employer-provided OHS.

The lack of OH provision, and particularly for workers in SMEs, has long been recognized. In 2008, a review by Dame Carol Black[15] recommended the government should pilot a new Fit for Work service based on case-managed, multidisciplinary support for patients in the early stages of sickness absence, with the aim of making access to work-related health support available to all. It also recommended the government initiate a business-led health and wellbeing consultancy service geared towards smaller organizations, offering tailored advice and support and access to occupational health support at a market rate.

Following pilots, the government duly launched a Fit for Work service[16] in December 2014, which was aimed primarily at SMEs and their workers. Fit for Work is delivered in England and Wales by Health Management, which is part of the MAXIMUS group, and in Scotland by the Scottish government as Fit for Work Scotland.[17] The service had two components, offering:

- GPs and employers the ability to refer a worker for a state-funded assessment of employees by occupational health professionals. To qualify for a referral, an employee must have been in paid employment, consented to the referral and not been referred to the service within the previous year; and

- free, expert and impartial advice on issues around health and work for workers employers and GPs[18] This comprises a helpline, webchat and email service with specialist advisers, as well as online resources.

Unfortunately, the government announced in November 2017 that it was scrapping the referral and assessment component of Fit for Work, which ceased in England and Wales at the end of March 2018 and in Scotland at the end of May 2018. The government blamed low referral rates and poor uptake of the service, although this may, at least in part, have been due to inadequate promotion of the scheme and engagement with employees, employers and GPs by the government.

In Scotland, some workers can now refer themselves to an NHS service, Working Health Services Scotland[19] if they are either:

- self-employed and struggling at work ('presenteeism') due to ill health or a condition, or are absent from work for any length of time; or

- an employee in a company with no more than 250 employees, are struggling at work due to ill health or a condition or are absent for no more than three weeks and do not have access to an OHS.

The service provides free, professional, confidential health and wellbeing assessments, support and advice. Where appropriate, it will refer workers to locally delivered treatments, including physiotherapy, occupational therapy and counselling. The workers are assigned a case manager who will:

- complete a comprehensive assessment;
- develop an action plan;
- coordinate treatment;
- liaise with the worker's GP, if required, and other relevant professionals; and
- suggest services for help and advice on issues such as housing, employment and debt management.

Employee Assistance Programmes

Many employees will have access to an Employee Assistance Programme (EAP), which is a service that can help you deal with personal problems that arise from work and non-work settings. The UK Employment Assistance Professionals Association, which represents EAP professionals, estimated that 13.79 million employees had access to an EAP in 2013, which would amount to 47% of the working population.[20] EAPs[21] are essentially counselling and advice services that should be no more than one part of your employer's approach to health and wellbeing. Crucially, they are not an alternative to your employer implementing organizational policies and preventive measures on mental health, stress and bullying.

If you have access to an EAP, it will usually be provided by an external organization and paid for by your employer, usually on the basis of the number of employees or use. This means that it is more feasible for SMEs to offer the service to their employees, although uptake among smaller firms is below that of larger organizations. Some larger employers will have their own internal EAP, but employees can be reluctant to use these services because they may perceive them as neither impartial nor confidential.

Typically, an EAP operates around the clock 365 days a year. It will offer telephone and online advice and face-to-face counselling although, as the TUC notes, the counselling is often restricted to a limited number of sessions, after which 'the EAP provider may try to get the employee to pay for further sessions privately or refer them to a commercial provider, even where free services may be available', for example through the NHS.[22]

The service is confidential, although the EAP may provide anonymized feedback to your employer on any common problems, for example if it was handling a number of bullying complaints. The EAP might liaise between the employee and a manager if there is a problem, although this obviously may give rise to issues of anonymity and confidentiality. The types of issue on which an EAP might provide advice are set out in the box. The EAP Association notes, however, that surveys show that:

EAPs are typically being used in a limited way – as the fallback option for staff who have a crisis. EAPs should be a major platform for supporting wellbeing and resilience in our new world of work, coaching people to feel better able to cope, to be happier and more productive.[23]

EAPs: what's on offer?

The types of issues about which an EAP may offer advice include:

- work-related problems, including bullying, harassment, problems with colleagues;
- stress;
- emotional problems;
- financial difficulties;
- legal issues;
- domestic issues;
- drug or alcohol abuse;
- life management skills.

Persuading your employer

If you employer is reluctant to use OH advice, it is worth reminding it that it has a duty under the Management of Health and Safety at Work Regulations 1999 to appoint one or more competent persons to assist it in complying with its health and safety duties. Competent persons must have sufficient training and experience or knowledge and other qualities to enable them to carry out their work. The SOM points out that: 'While a health professional is not always needed, employers still need to call on an appropriately qualified doctor or nurse to deal with any work-related health problems.' The Regulations also require your employer to ensure that you and your colleagues are provided with health surveillance as appropriate to the risks.

Statutory duties aside, there a great deal of evidence to show that using an OHS can benefit you, your employer and the wider economy. The Society of Occupational Medicine (SOM) has published an analysis of the evidence of the value of OHSs, which suggested that it is important to make a broad business case of the value of OH that goes beyond economic return on investment to incorporate wide-ranging and sometimes intangible factors.[24] It found that employers commission OH services mainly to enhance performance and to ensure compliance with regulations or policy. Moreover, 'the moral case' is particularly important among smaller organizations and that it is therefore 'necessary to present OH services as affordable and cost effective to organizations and good for their business'.

Notes

1 Campaign details: www.whyoccupationalhealth.co.uk/content/ why-occupational-health

2 SOM (2017) OH: *a guide for workers and their representatives,* www.whyoccupationalhealth.co.uk/sites/all/themes/zen/uploads/ Occupational%20health%20-%20A%20guide%20for%20 workers%20and%20their%20representatives.pdf

3 Department for Work and Pensions, *Getting the most out of the fit note. Guidance for employers and line managers,* assets. publishing.service.gov.uk/government/uploads/system/uploads/ attachment_data/file/578032/fit-note-guidance-for-employers-and-line-managers.pdf

4 NHS Digital (2017) *Fit notes issued by GP practices, England. December 2014–March 2017* digital.nhs.uk/catalogue/PUB30068

5 TUC (2016) *Medical referrals in employment – is the doctor appropriately qualified?*, www.tuc.org.uk/research-analysis/ reports/medical-referrals-employment—-doctor-appropriately-qualified

6 bit.ly/2HDIHDH

7 TUC (2016) *Medical referrals in employment*

8 TUC (2016) *Is my OH provider accredited?* www.tuc.org.uk/ research-analysis/reports/my-occupational-health-provider-accredited

9 SEQOHS accredited services: www.seqohs.org/Accreditedunits. aspx

10 DWP (2011) *Health and wellbeing at work: a survey of employees'*, Research Report no.751, bit.ly/2h5vwgy

11 Black C (2016) *Working for a healthier tomorrow: work and health in Britain 2008*, bit.ly/2HGgU5B

12 All Party Parliamentary Group on Occupational Safety and Health (2016) *Occupational medical workforce crisis. The need for action to keep the UK workforce healthy*, https:// d3n8a8pro7vhmx.cloudfront.net/ianlavery/pages/150/ attachments/original/1476691067/OM_Workforce_Crisis_2016_ pdf.pdf?1476691067

13 Faculty of Occupational Medicine (2011) *The future need for specialist occupational physicians in the UK*, www.fom.ac.uk/ wp-content/uploads/FOM-Recruitment-of-specialist-OPs-in-UK-August-2011.pdf; Council for Work and Health (2016), *Planning the future. Implications for OH delivery and training*, www. councilforworkandhealth.org.uk/images/uploads/library/ Final%20Report%20-%20Planning%20the%20Future%20-%20Implications%20for%20OH%20-%20Proof%202.pdf

14 GMC (2014) *The state of medical education and practice in the UK.* www.gmc-uk.org/-/media/documents/SOMEP_2014_FINAL. pdf_58751753.pdf

15 Black C (2008) *Working for a healthier tomorrow*

16 Fit for Work service: www.orwork.org. government guidance on the service: www.gov.uk/government/collections/fit-for-work-guidance

17 fitforworkscotland.scot, or tel: 0800 019 2211

18 fitforwork.org. Tel: 0800 032 6235 (English) or 0800 032 6233 (Cymraeg)

19 0800 019 2211

20 EAP Association (2013) *EAP 2013 market watch*, www.eapa.org. uk/wp-content/uploads/2014/02/UK-EAPA-MARKET-WATCH-REPORT-2013.pdf

21 A list of EAP providers is at: www.eapa.org.uk/find-an-eap-provider

22 TUC (2013) *Work and wellbeing*, www.tuc.org.uk/sites/default/files/tucfiles/TUC_WORK_AND_WELL-BEING.pdf

23 EAP Association (2013) *The evolution of employee assistance: investigating the use, impact and reach of EAPs in today's organisations*, www.eapa.org.uk/wp-content/uploads/2014/02/UK-EAPA-Reseach-Report-The-evolution-of-employee-assistance-FINAL.pdf

24 SOM (2017) *OH: the value proposition*, www.som.org.uk/sites/som.org.uk/files/Occupational%20health%20-%20the%20value%20proposition.pdf

Chapter 13
New ways of working

The world of work is changing. Whether it's zero-hours contracts, insecure work or the gig economy,[1] these new ways of working come with a range of health risks. And while there's no simple solution, researchers, trade unions, workers and politicians have many good ideas to help make these jobs more healthy.

New work

The way we work is changing. More than three million people – that's one in 10 of the UK workforce – now face insecurity at work. Not only do they often face uncertainty about their working hours, they also miss out on rights and protections that many of us take for granted, from being able to return to the same job after having a baby to the right to sick pay when they can't work.[2]

When it comes to zero-hours, 1.4 million contracts don't guarantee a minimum number of hours according to the ONS's twice yearly survey of businesses, and the Labour Force Survey found that 883,000 people – almost 3% of the workforce – were employed on zero-hours contracts in their main job between April and June 2017. People on zero-hours contracts are more likely to be young, part-time, women or in full-time education compared with other people in employment. Those on zero-hours contracts work 26 hours a week on average, and 26.6% would like more hours, compared with just 7.2% of other people in employment.[3]

New technology has also produced new models of work – and these are spreading to new areas of work. A survey by the RSA (Royal Society for the encouragement of Arts, Manufactures and Commerce) found that 59% of gig workers provide professional and administrative services, 33% skilled manual or professional services and 16% driving or delivery services.[4] Mobile apps and online platforms make it easy to connect workers with customers, and although gig economy companies operate in parts of the economy that traditionally relied on self-employed workers, new technology is changing things in a such rapid and far-reaching way that there are now around 1.1 million people working in the gig economy in the UK.

Not surprisingly, the number of people who are self-employed or on zero-hour contracts is increasing. In London, for example, levels of self-employment have risen by 38% over the past 10 years and 2.5% of London's working population are on zero-hours contracts.[5]

The numbers are significant, but the reasons why people work in the gig economy are even more important. You'll often see flexibility and choice being highlighted as major benefits of gig work. However, government figures and other surveys show that up to one third of people do this kind of work because they cannot get regular employment.[6]

The modern economy

In response to these major changes, in 2016 the Prime Minister Theresa May commissioned an independent review of employment practices in the modern economy from Matthew Taylor, the chief executive of the RSA. Published a year later the report, *Good work*, said that despite record levels of employment in the UK, the quantity of work needs to be matched by its quality. It called on the government to 'adopt the ambition that all work should be fair and decent'.[7]

The report says that good work matters because bad work – work that is insecure, exploitative, and/or controlling – is bad for health and wellbeing, and it calls for more concerted efforts to improve the quality of work in the economy. Although there's no single index or set of data on quality of work, it's generally agreed that quality depends on several things, including pay, working conditions, terms of employment, health and safety, work-life balance, and whether or not you have representation or a way to make your voice heard at work. The TUC's *Great Jobs Agenda* report argues that these are all preconditions for a happy and satisfying working life.

To improve the quality of work, the report called on the government to simplify the UK's confusing mixture of different categories of employment by aligning employment law with tax regulations. These complex, overlapping categories have made it easy for gig employers to deny workers rights to sick pay etc, and there have been several high-profile court cases where plumbers, Uber drivers and Deliveroo riders have gone to court to fight for rights for themselves and for others (see box).

The report also talked about flexibility, saying that while mutual flexibility is a good thing, one-sided 'flexibility' that suits only the employer must be tackled. 'One sided flexibility is when employers seek to transfer all risk on to the shoulders of workers in ways which make people more insecure and make their lives harder to manage,' it said.

And as well as drawing clearer boundaries between who is a worker and who is self-employed, the report also said what employers do to support health and wellbeing at work should be recognized and supported (see chapter 11).

The three-tier workforce

In the UK, your rights vary a lot depending on your employment status. Under current UK employment law there are three main types of employment status: employee, worker, and self-employed or contractor.[8] The self-employed have few rights at work. These include health and safety protections and protection from discrimination in some circumstances.

People classified as 'workers' fare slightly better, and have the right to be paid the national minimum wage, holiday pay, working time protections, protection from discrimination and some union rights. However, core protections including job security rights, family-friendly rights and protection from arbitrary treatment are reserved for 'employees', who also tend to be entitled to benefits associated with stable employment, such as enhanced sick pay and pensions. People engaged in more 'flexible' forms of work bear all the risk. Their employment can be terminated at a moment's notice, they have no guaranteed hours and are not entitled to redundancy pay if work dries up.[9]

As a result, plumbers, Uber drivers, Deliveroo riders and others have gone to court – with the help of trade unions like the GMB and the Independent Workers' Union of Great Britain – to fight for their rights. Many of these cases have involved deciding whether people working in the gig economy are workers or self-employed.[10]

You can find out more about these court cases at www.gmb.org.uk and https://iwgb.org.uk

Why poor quality work is bad for your health

The gig economy might be a relatively new way of working, but there is good evidence that insecure, poor quality work is bad for your health.

A large study of more than 7,000 young adults found that people on zero-hours contracts were less likely to be in good health – and were at higher risk of poor mental health – than those with stable jobs. The analysis is part of a long-running study called Next Steps, which was set up by the government in 2004 to track millennials from school and into work and is now run by UCL's Institute of Education. The study's lead author

Dr Morag Henderson said that zero-hours contracts could be affecting people's mental and physical health because of the stress that goes along with this way of working. As well as its impact on mental health, the financial stress and worry associated with irregular work could also be causing physical symptoms such as headaches and muscle tension, she said.[11]

A recent IOSH-commissioned survey of 500 non-permanent workers found that only one third had access to occupational health support (compared with 54% of their permanent colleagues), 43% had no holiday pay and one quarter worked unpaid overtime. Two thirds did not receive sick pay, and half of these said that to make sure that they got paid, they worked when they were sick. One person said they'd been sent into work by their employer despite suffering from the winter vomiting bug norovirus, which is extremely unpleasant and very easy to spread to other people.[12]

A survey commissioned by the London Assembly's health committee also found big differences in access to health support between low and higher-paid employees. Low paid employees were much more fearful of talking to their employer about a health condition, and much less likely to have access to regular health checks through their employers.

Only 4% of lowest paid employees with a health condition said they had tried talking to their manager about it, compared with 22% of the highest paid employees. On health support, 40% of the highest paying employers provide regular health checks, compared with 16% of the lowest paying employers. And only 40% of low paid employees think that their employer would support them if they needed time off for a mental illness, compared with 59% of higher paid employees.[13]

Long hours, lone working and stress

There are lots of ways in which insecure work can negatively affect your physical and mental health. Many of these relate to the ingredients that affect the quality of work, which we discussed earlier in this book.

Quality work is strongly linked to better health outcomes for individuals. As the Taylor report shows, good work not only enables people to support themselves and their families financially but with the right kind of support, from employers and others, work has a positive impact on health and well-being.[14]

The opposite is true of insecure work. Low pay and zero-hours force many people to work long hours in several jobs just to make ends meet. It's not unusual for people to work shifts in one kind of job – in retail or the hospitality industry, for example – followed by several hours driving for a delivery or ride-sharing firm.

Working long hours affects your health in lots of ways. Working while you're tired means you're at greater risk of accidents. Being awake for 24 hours, say sleep experts, impairs your performance to the same degree as being over the drink driving limit. Sleep disruption also affects our emotions and mental health.[15] And long hours also make it harder to eat well, get enough exercise, and relax with your family and friends – all things that we need to stay healthy (see chapters 9 and 11).

Insecure work is also stressful. This might be because of the pace or intensity of work. You might be afraid of losing your job (for example because of the ratings systems some gig employers ask their customers to use), or not knowing from one day to the next how many hours you'll be working. In a GMB survey of 1,000 people in precarious employment, six out of 10 said their current job was causing them stress or anxiety.[16] Many studies show that the less control you have over your work, the greater the stress, and if your hours are not guaranteed, you are more likely to work long hours when they're offered. These kind of employment relationships also make it harder for people to report unsafe or unhealthy working conditions.

We've seen that young workers and women are more likely to work in the gig economy. Added to this, gig work often involves working outside, at night, in all weathers, or on your own in someone else's house. These are all environments that increase health and safety risks (see chapter 14).

Lastly, working on your own poses additional problems. Many of the health benefits of work – particularly for mental health – come from working together with colleagues. And working alone makes it hard to have a voice at work and to join a trade union, which is important because trade union safety representatives help make their workplaces safer and healthier.[17]

Healthier work?

Since the publication of *Good work*, there's been a significant amount of debate in government, trade unions and health and safety organizations about how to make new ways of working healthier. Making progress depends on action from many quarters.

Good work – the review of modern working practices that the government commissioned – made seven key recommendations. Good work and plentiful work can and should go together, it said, adding that 'good work is something for which government needs to be held accountable but for which we all need to take responsibility'. Workers – or 'dependent contractors' as the report would like to see them called – should have additional protection and there should be stronger incentives for firms to treat them fairly. On health at work, the report said that because work has such a strong impact on health, there needs to be a 'more proactive approach to workplace health'.[18]

The London Assembly's report *Work and health* said that we need to challenge the idea that there will always be some bad or unhealthy jobs. It made some specific suggestions about how to make new ways of working more healthy, including more dialogue between employers and workers, better education and more representation.

Employers need greater understanding of their workers' experiences so that they can develop more effective strategies, and people need to be more informed about healthy work so that they can have constructive conversations with their employers, the report said. It asked the Mayor of London to use a programme called Healthy Schools London to teach young people about healthy and unhealthy work so that they leave school better equipped to challenge unhealthy work practices. And the report called on the Mayor to talk to Public Health England about roving health and work champions for small employers.[19]

Although we know that insecure work is bad for health, we still need good quality data about working in the gig economy – from the hazards people face to their impact on health. From the 1960s to the 1980s, thousands of civil servants were studied in order to unpick the effects of pay grade on stress and heart disease. Known as the Whitehall studies, they provided valuable evidence of the links between stress and autonomy at work. Dr Chris Yuill, head of sociology at Robert Gordon University in Aberdeen, says it's time we invested in a 'Gighall' study.[20]

Having more data on work and health in low-paid workers in the hospitality sector, for example, is also something the London Assembly wants to see, and its report said that the Mayor should commission research to fill this gap.[21]

Evidence from other countries suggests that there is nothing inevitable about insecurity in the modern world of work. The TUC argues that we can tackle insecurity by increasing unions' ability to negotiate better terms and conditions in their workplace, updating the framework of employment rights to protect everyone, improving the enforcement of those rights, and ensuring that our tax and social security systems both incentivize secure jobs, and protect those currently facing insecurity.[22]

Responding to *Good work*, in February 2018 the government announced that it would give gig economy workers new rights, including holiday and sick pay, for the first time, as well as giving all workers the right to demand a payslip, and allowing flexible workers to demand more stable contracts. It will also monitor and report on the quality as well as the quantity of jobs in the economy and take steps to make sure flexible workers are aware of their rights.

But many, including the TUC, say these changes don't go far enough. According to TUC general secretary Frances O'Grady: 'The government has taken a baby step – when it needed to take a giant leap. These plans won't stop the hire and fire culture of zero-hours contracts or sham self-employment. And they will still leave 1.8 million workers excluded from key protections.'

How long it takes for our employment laws to catch up with these new ways of working remains to be seen. The issue will not go away but eventually campaigns and court cases should bring change.

Notes

1 *gig economy*: 'a labour market characterized by the prevalence of short-term contracts or freelance work as opposed to permanent jobs' (Oxford Dictionaries)

2 TUC. *The gig is up*. www.tuc.org.uk/sites/default/files/the-gig-is-up.pdf

3 ONS (2017) Contracts that do not guarantee a minimum number of hours. www.ons.gov.uk/employmentandlabourmarket/peopleinwork/earningsandworkinghours/articles/contractsthatdonotguaranteeaminimumnumberofhours/september2017

4 RSA (2017) Good gigs: A fairer future for the UK's gig economy. www.thersa.org/globalassets/pdfs/reports/rsa_good-gigs-fairer-gig-economy-report.pdf

5 London Assembly (2018) *Work and health*. www.london.gov.uk/sites/default/files/work_and_health_findings_report_final_formatted.pdf

6 CIPD (2017) *To gig or not to gig? Stories from the modern economy*. www.cipd.co.uk/Images/to-gig-or-not-to-gig_2017-stories-from-the-modern-economy_tcm18-18955.pdf

7 HM government (2017) *Good work: The Taylor review of modern working practices*. www.gov.uk/government/uploads/system/uploads/attachment_data/file/627671/good-work-taylor-review-modern-working-practices-rg.pdf

8 See www.gov.uk/employment-status

9 TUC (2017) *The gig is up*

10 House of Lords (2018) *Gig economy: Legal status of gig economy workers and working practices*. http://researchbriefings.files.parliament.uk/documents/LLN-2018-0026/LLN-2018-0026.pdf

11 UCL Institute of Education (2017) *Economic activity and health: Initial findings from the Next Steps* Age 25 Sweep. www.cls.ioe.ac.uk/shared/get-file.ashx?itemtype=document&id=3301

12 IOSH (2017) www.iosh.co.uk/News/Survey-of-gig-workers-health-and-wellbeing.aspx

13 London Assembly (2018) *Health and work*

14 HM government (2017) *Good work*

15 Lockley SW and Foster R (2012) *Sleep: A very short introduction*, OUP

16 GMB (2017) www.gmb.org.uk/newsroom/millions-insecure-work

17 TUC (2016) *The union effect*. www.tuc.org.uk/research-analysis/reports/union-effect

18 HM government (2017) *Good work*

19 London Assembly (2018) *Health and work*

20 Ahuja A (2017) 'Why 'gig health' matters', *Financial Times*, 25 May. www.ft.com/content/bdc90c22-408f-11e7-82b6-896b95f30f58

21 London Assembly (2018) *Health and work*

22 TUC (2017) *The gig is up*

Chapter 14
Young or inexperienced workers and apprentices

As a young worker, you are an essential part of the workforce and should, with help and supervision, be no more likely than your older colleagues to suffer health and wellbeing problems. In fact, your youth will help you avoid some aches and pains. You may, however, face risks that can arise from inexperience and being new to the workplace. As such, you and your union representatives need to make sure that you have the confidence and help from your employer that you need to do your job and stay healthy. Staying healthy will help you become one of tomorrow's supervisors, or a mentor, manager or director. You will then be able to help safeguard the next generations of young workers and help them to instil the good habits that you learned. With the numbers of apprentices set to treble by 2020, safeguarding the mental and physical health of young workers has become more pressing than ever.

Young workers can be particularly vulnerable to harm through a lack of experience and expertise, poor awareness of occupational risks and a lack of physical and/or psychological maturity.[1] Someone new to the world of work may also be particularly keen to impress their colleagues and managers – no bad thing, unless it leads you to take on a task that should be left alone, or attempt something beyond your training and experience level. And while there are no indications that young workers 'fool around' any more than their older colleagues, you can be at risk from employers giving you tasks without providing sufficient information, instruction, supervision and training.

Contrary to some perceptions, workers aged 16–24 take fewer days off work for, and have the lowest rates of, work-related illnesses than any other age group.[2] Such statistics, however, may not tell the full story. There is often a long period – sometimes decades – between exposure to a hazard and the appearance of ill-health symptoms, for example developing mesothelioma from asbestos exposure. Other conditions are cumulative and may require exposure over a period of time, for example from vibrating tools, before symptoms appear. It is often difficult to focus on a possible consequence that may not manifest for many years, if at all, but it is vital that young workers take account of such potential exposures from day one.

As a young worker, the law will either prevent you from working with many hazardous substances and in high-risk situations, or it will require your employer to ensure that you carry out the work only under strict supervision and controls. You will also have the advantage that your bodies will not have been subject to years of wear and tear, which can lead to or exacerbate ill-health conditions.

Injury statistics, on first viewing, point similarly to a lower rate among young workers. Research from the Health and Safety Executive (HSE) and the European Agency for Safety and Health at Work, however, found that if allowances are made for the types of occupations and characteristics of the job, male workers aged 16–24 have a 40% higher risk than their 45–54-year-old colleagues of being injured at work.[3] This does not mean you are automatically at increased risk, just that you, your colleagues and your representatives need to make sure you have the safeguards that are appropriate to the type of work you are doing.

The legal protections

If you are a young worker – essentially, if you are under 18 years of age – you are covered by the same health and safety legislation as any other worker, but you will also have some additional safeguards in law. The Management of Health and Safety at Work Regulations 1999 prohibit employers from employing young persons unless they have carried out or reviewed their risk assessment to take account of:

- the inexperience, lack of awareness of risks and immaturity of young persons;
- the fitting-out and layout of the workplace and the workstation;
- the nature, degree and duration of exposure to physical, biological and chemical agents;
- the form, range, and use of work equipment and the way in which it is handled;
- the organization of processes and activities;
- the health and safety training provided to young persons; and
- risks from physical, biological and chemical agents, processes and work listed in the young workers Directive 94/33/EC, for example lead, asbestos and work involving high-voltage electricity or structural collapse.

This list means that employers must specifically ensure that young persons are protected from any risks to their health or safety that are a consequence of their lack of experience, risk awareness or maturity. In certain work circumstances, they are also prohibited from employing young workers at all, unless three conditions are met: the work must be necessary for the young person's training; the young person will be supervised by a competent person; and the risk must be reduced to the lowest level that is reasonably practicable. These restrictions apply when the work involves:

- tasks that are beyond the young person's physical or psychological capacity;
- harmful exposure to agents that are toxic, carcinogenic, cause heritable genetic damage or harm to an unborn child or that in any other way chronically affects health;
- harmful exposure to radiation;
- a risk of accidents that a young person cannot recognize or avoid because of insufficient attention to safety or lack of experience or training; or
- a risk to health from extreme cold or heat, noise or vibration.

The Working Time Regulations 1998 also give young persons specific protection against excessive working hours and insufficient breaks. Under these Regulations, young persons must have:

- a 30-minute daily rest break when working for more than four and a half hours (adults are entitled to 20 minutes where the work is more than six hours);
- a daily rest period of 12 consecutive hours in any 24-hour period (11 consecutive hours for adult workers); and
- a weekly rest period of 48 hours (consecutive where possible) in every seven-day period (24 hours for adult workers).

All workers – young and adult – have the same entitlements to a maximum 48-hour working week and to 28 days of paid annual leave each year (including bank holidays). All night workers must not work for more than an average of eight hours in any 24-hour period. The reference period for adult night workers is 11pm to 6am. Young workers, however, are also prohibited from working between 10pm and 6am unless they have had a health assessment before starting the work and at regular intervals thereafter.

What to do?

There is a great deal of guidance on young workers and apprentices, including from the TUC[4] and individual trade unions, the Royal Society for the Prevention of Accidents (RoSPA, which carried out an inquiry into apprentices in 2016 and 2017),[5] the British Safety Council,[6] employers' bodies such as the EEF,[7] and from the HSE. Fortunately, there is significant consensus as to what constitutes employer good practice when applying the legislation.

Employers and trade unions in general find young persons willing to learn and take instruction, and interested in protecting their health and safety. Young persons will, however, have had vastly different learning experiences from older workers. They may, for example, be more accustomed to using the internet to find out information instantaneously.

Drawing on this, young workers and their union representatives should check:

- the risk assessment that employers are required to carry out covers all aspects of the work of a young person or apprentice before they start work, and that it takes account of the traits and risks that may be pertinent to young persons;
- the risk assessment and arrangements take account of any young persons with learning difficulties and/or disabilities. In 2016/17, 10% (50,500) of persons starting an apprenticeship had learning difficulties and/or disabilities, up from 26,400 in 2009/10. Although the increase as a proportion of all apprentices is less significant, the total number of young persons with learning difficulties and/or

disabilities on apprenticeships is likely to increase as part of the overall increase in apprenticeships;

- training – both at induction and subsequently – covers health, wellbeing and safety and the work that the young person will be performing, and that the training is monitored;

- supervisors and mentors are trained, competent and provided with sufficient time to supervise a young person, and that there are sufficient numbers of supervisors, mentors and competent colleagues to help young workers;

- young workers receive appropriate personal protective equipment and instruction in how to use it;

- analysis of work-related illnesses and injuries looks at young workers and apprentices as a separate category;

- the complexity and risks of tasks is increased gradually;

- ensure that the ways of learning are appropriate – a case study of an injury or statistical risks of developing an asbestos-related disease can grab a young person's attention but it can also be worrying if not explained properly;

- the young worker is able and empowered to raise concerns; and

- there are regular reviews carried out by internal and external teams.

It is also important to persuade employers to consider health and wellbeing away from the workplace. This is important for all employees but particularly so for young workers and apprentices, many of whom will be living away from home with incomes for the first time. A holistic approach should extend to alcohol and drug abuse, debt and mental health issues. Are you, or your young colleagues, aware of any employee assistance programmes or equivalent that your employer might offer? Explain too the mutual benefits of investing in additional driver training for young workers: drivers aged between 17 and 24 hold 7% of UK driving licences but are involved in 22% of fatal or serious collisions.[8]

Some of these challenges may be exacerbated in smaller firms because of a lack of competent staff, work pressures, and a lack of health and safety knowledge. Conversely, the closer relationships engendered in some small firms can result in greater vigilance for their young charges.

Apprentices

If the government realizes its targets, the number of apprentices in England will increase from 912,200 in 2016/17[9] to three million by 2020, which will have implications for safeguarding the health and wellbeing of young workers. As we note elsewhere in the book, young workers account for a significant proportion of apprenticeships: in 2016/17, 25% of starts were aged 18 or below, and 29% were aged 19–24, with 46% among workers aged 25 and over. These proportions have been generally consistent since 2011/12. (Before 2004/05, apprenticeships were not available for people over the age of 24.)

A new Apprentice Levy, which started in May 2017, requires all UK employers with an annual pay bill that exceeds £3 million to pay 0.5% of the wage bill into a fund, which the government tops up by 10%. The employers can only spend the fund on apprenticeship training costs. The government also pays 90% of training costs for organizations that fall outside of the levy, and makes some additional payments for young workers.

Worryingly for the government, the 491,300 apprenticeship starts during 2016/17 was 18,100 fewer than in 2015/16. Moreover, the drop was particularly marked in the final quarter (May to July) of 2016/17, with 130,000 fewer starts than in the corresponding quarter a year earlier. The government attributed the drop to changes in funding changes and the levy, with the minister of state at the Department of Education, Anne Milton, insisting that it was 'only natural that employers, and the apprenticeship market, take time to reflect on what the changes mean and how to maximise the opportunities they represent'.[10]

A large amount of information on health and wellbeing appears targeted at apprentices in sectors such as construction and allied trades. It is worth remembering, however, that almost 9 in 10 starts in 2016/17 were in four sectors: health, public services and care (138,000 starts in 2016/17 and 44,000 starts in 2009/10); business, administration and the law (137,000 and 77,000); retail and commercial enterprise (75,000 and 62,000); and engineering and manufacturing technologies (74,000 and 43,000). The numbers of apprentices in construction, planning and the built environment were 21,000 in both years.

Training providers

Although employers have the principal duty to ensure your health and safety as an apprentice, training providers and placement organizers must also do their part, with failures to do so graphically illustrated in the tragic death of Cameron Minshull (see box). The HSE's website offers guidance on young workers[11] for schools and colleges, work experience organizers,[12] placement providers, parents and carers, and students and learners. The HSE advises training providers that while they do not have to 'second guess' an employer's risk assessment and control measures, they nonetheless have to take reasonable steps that are 'in proportion to the environment' to satisfy themselves that the employer is doing this. The interpretation of reasonable can be problematic, with the RoSPA inquiry finding training providers unclear as to the difference between the three levels of interaction with employers suggested by the HSE.

Depending on the level and nature of the risk, the HSE reminds training providers that they must satisfy themselves as to what you will be doing and that the risk management arrangements are adequate by:

- speaking to employers in low-risk environments, such as offices or shops, with everyday risks that will mostly be familiar to the apprentice;

- talking to employers in environments that have less familiar risks, for example light assembly or packing facilities; or

- discussing with employers in higher-risk environments such as construction, agriculture or manufacturing.

CASE STUDY The Death of Cameron Minshull

Cameron Minshull started work on 3 December 2012 on a government-funded Skills Training Agency apprenticeship at Huntley Mount Engineering in Manchester. He was killed just 36 days later after he was pulled inside a Computerised Numeric Control lathe while 'deburring' components with an emery cloth. He had been carrying out this work by putting his arm inside the running machine. He was aged 16.

The investigation by the Greater Manchester Police (GMP) and the Health and Safety Executive (HSE) found that the lathe's interlock had been disabled, as had safety features on the company's other lathes, and that the company's other young employees used the same method that killed Mr Minshull. There were no risk assessments, no meaningful supervision and the training was inadequate, with the company's sole director and supervisor telling the apprentices to roll up their sleeves.

On 14 July 2015, at Manchester Crown Court, Judge David Stockdale fined Huntley £150,000 for the corporate manslaughter of Mr Minshull.

The judge also imprisoned the firm's sole director, Zaffar Hussain, for eight months and disqualified him as a company director for 10 years for a breach of the Health and Safety at Work Act 1974. Judge Stockdale imposed a suspended four-month custodial term and a £3,000 fine on the firm's supervisor, Akbar Hussain, under the 1974 Act. The judge said the failures meant that the young apprentices were 'oblivious' to the risks from using an emery cloth and had been 'effectively left to their own devices'.

Judge Stockdale also fined Lime People Training Solutions, the company that placed Mr Minshull with Huntley, £75,000 for an offence under the 1974 Act. The company is now in liquidation. The investigation had found that that Lime People Training Solutions had placed Mr Minshull without carrying out 'even basic' health and safety checks that would, according to the Crown Prosecution Service, have shown it that Huntley was 'a wholly unsuitable placement' and that the system of work was 'grossly unsafe'. GMP's Inspector Ben Cottam said the case was 'a chilling reminder of the dangers of placing apprentices in potentially dangerous work environments'.

Notes

1 HSE (2015) *Employers perceptions of the health and safety of young workers*. HSE research report no.1061, bit.ly/1gozH2m

2 See, for example, HSE data sets WRIAGE1, WRIAGE2, WRIAGE3, bit.ly/1NV2746

3 OSHA (2009) *Preventing risks to young workers: policy, programmes and workplace practices*. bit.ly/1WHwnRI

4 TUC (2009) *Apprenticeships are union businesses*. bit.ly/1SL37og

5 RoSPA advice on young workers: bit.ly/1SZpaNs

6 See British Safety Council (BSC) advice on young workers ('Speak up. Stay safe'): bit.ly/21tp0Ov and BSC (2010),'*Ensuring the safety and health of young workers*, bit.ly/1Y65zth

7 EEF bit.ly/1W4Nrls

8 RoSPA, *Young drivers*, www.rospa.com/resources/hubs/young-drivers

9 Andy Powell, *Apprenticeship statistics: England*, House of Commons Briefing Paper, No.06113, 15 December 2017, researchbriefings.files.parliament.uk/documents/SN06113/SN06113.pdf

10 *Hansard*, written questions, 21 November 2017, no.112477, www.parliament.uk/written-questions-answers-statements/written-question/commons/2017-11-13/112477

11 See HSE (2013) *Young people at work*, bit.ly/1SLzXFy and HSE (2013), *Apprentices*, bit.ly/1Z90mku

12 HSE (2013) *Young people and work experience*, INDG364, www.hse.gov.uk/pubns/indg364.pdf

Chapter 15
Accommodating specific conditions

Many people of working age have one or more long-term health conditions. These include asthma, cancer, chronic fatigue syndrome or ME, brain injury, stroke, cardiovascular disease, neurological conditions such as Parkinson's disease, epilepsy and migraine, diabetes, depression, chronic pain and musculoskeletal conditions. How much impact they have on your work depends on many things, including the support you get from your employer.

Although these conditions are very different, they can affect people's ability to work in similar ways. These can be due to symptoms like fatigue or pain, they can be disability-related such as poor mobility and dexterity, or they can result from people's working environment and employers' attitudes.

This chapter focuses on four long-term conditions or diseases – epilepsy, diabetes, migraine and cancer. These are all very different, but because they can have similar impacts on work, they illustrate how we can make workplaces better for people with all sorts of long-term conditions.[1] You can find out more about other long-term conditions at work in the information section at the end of the chapter and from your occupational health service (see chapter 14).

About migraine

Migraine is often described as a severe headache, but for people with migraine it can be a debilitating condition which has a major impact on work and family life. Migraine affects around 8 million people in the UK (that's one in seven of us), but despite the fact it's the most common neurological condition in the developed world, it remains misunderstood, stigmatized and under-managed.[2]

Migraine is a complex condition and symptoms vary. For many, a painful headache is the main symptom, but there can also be visual disturbances (eg aura, tunnel vision, blind spots), nausea, vomiting, and sensitivity to light, noise and smells. The duration and frequency of attacks also varies. Attacks can last from 4 to 72 hours and most people have no symptoms between attacks, and while some people have migraine attacks only once or twice a year, others have them two or three times a week.[3]

Migraine affects more women than men, usually begins early in life and although the underlying cause is uncertain, experts think there is a genetic cause which – given certain triggers – makes nerves in the brain malfunction. Many people's migraine attacks are brought on by certain triggers. These also vary, but common triggers include missing meals, dehydration, irregular sleep patterns, stress, travel and levels of the hormone oestrogen in women – which is why a woman's periods, childbirth and menopause can all affect her migraine.[4]

Why migraine is a workplace issue

Migraine is a workplace issue because of the impact it has on individuals and their employers. People with migraine are often stigmatized at work, or their headaches trivialized.

Around 25 million working days are lost each year in the UK to due to migraine, yet many employers don't understand migraine and how debilitating it can be. According to a 2017 YouGov survey in 2017 by three UK migraine charities, 64% of people said that employers don't understand enough about migraine and its effects on their staff and 70% didn't know whether migraine can be classed as a disability.[5]

Under the Equality Act 2010, migraine may be considered as a disability if it has a substantially adverse and long-term effect on your ability to carry out normal day-to-day activities. The Act protects you from unlawful discrimination at all stages of the employment – from recruitment and employment conditions to dismissal and redundancy – and requires employers to make 'reasonable adjustments' (see box).

Supporting people with migraine at work

There are many things that migraine sufferers and their employers can do to help manage the condition at work. For individuals, the first question you'll face is whether – or when – to tell your employer. This can be daunting, particularly because of the stigma and misunderstanding surrounding migraine. There are good reasons, however, to talk to your employer. It will help raise awareness about migraine at work and, says the Migraine Trust, employers will be better able to provide appropriate support if they know that you have migraine attacks.

Many simple workplace changes can make a difference to migraine sufferers; these include employers' sickness absence policies, tackling migraine triggers, and making sure you look after yourself:

- Sickness absence: because migraine attacks can last between 4 and 72 hours, you're more likely to take short-term sickness absence. Check that your employer's sickness absence policy distinguishes between general sickness and absence due to disabilities such as migraine.

- Tackling triggers: this includes the physical environment such as having good lighting, using lamps with daylight bulbs rather than fluorescent lighting, reducing glare from windows and shiny surfaces, maintaining a comfortable temperature, reducing the volume of background music, and installing extractors to remove strong smells, and psychosocial factors, such as reducing workplace stress (see chapter 2).

- Looking after yourself: missing meals and dehydration can trigger migraine attacks, so remember to take breaks so that you can eat and drink enough.

- Awareness training: by providing information and training, employers can help raise awareness and reduce the stigma associated with migraine, both of which will help create a more supportive working environment.[6]

All these things are examples of good practice, but if the severity of your migraine means it's classed as a disability under the Equality Act 2010, your employer has a legal duty to make these kinds of 'reasonable adjustment'.

Equality Act 2010

If you live and work in the UK, the law protects you from discrimination at work. The Equality Act 2010 applies in England, Scotland and Wales (with the exception of the armed forces). Different legislation applies in Northern Ireland.[7] As far as health at work is concerned, the Equality Act is important because it covers people with disabilities.

The Act defines disability as any physical or mental impairment which has a substantially adverse and long-term effect on your ability to carry out normal day-to-day activities. That means that even if you don't think that your migraine, epilepsy or other long-term health condition is a disability, the law might do so, and therefore protect you against discrimination. If you have cancer, HIV or Multiple Sclerosis, the Act considers you as disabled from the point of diagnosis.

Being covered by the Act means that your employer must consider making 'reasonable adjustments' if they are aware of your disability, if you ask for adjustments or if you're having difficulty with your work.

You can find out more about disability discrimination and legal rights at:

Acas – the workplace relationships and employment law experts – and health charities such as Macmillan Cancer Support and Diabetes UK publish free guidance on the Equality Act.

Acas Disability discrimination: key points for the workplace. www.acas.org.uk/index.aspx?articleid=1859

Diabetes UK (2017). *Employment and diabetes: advocacy pack.* www.diabetes.org.uk/resources-s3/2017-09/Advocacy%20pack_EmploymentV3-Jan2016_0.pdf

Macmillan Cancer Support. *Legal rights about work and cancer*: www.macmillan.org.uk/information-and-support/organising/work-and-cancer/if-youre-an-employer/legislation-about-work-and-cancer.html

Equality Commission (2011). *Disability discrimination law in NI: a short guide.* www.equalityni.org/ECNI/media/ECNI/Publications/Individuals/DisabilityDiscrimShortGuide2011.pdf?ext=.pdf

About epilepsy

If you've been diagnosed with epilepsy, you are not alone. Around 600,000 people in the UK have epilepsy, making it one of the most common long-term ill-health conditions in the workplace. It can start at any age, but is most commonly diagnosed before the age of 20 or when you're over 65.

Epilepsy can be caused by a specific event, like a head injury, but it can also begin suddenly and doctors may be unable to discover why. It's not necessarily a life-long diagnosis; if you have been free of seizures for long enough, doctors may consider that you no longer have epilepsy.

Epilepsy simply means that you have a tendency to have epileptic seizures, which some people call 'fits' or 'attacks'. Seizures occur when there's a sudden, intense burst of electrical activity in the brain, which temporarily disrupts the way the brain works.

What happens during a seizure depends on where in the brain the disruption begins, and how widely and rapidly it spreads. As a result, there are many different types of seizure and your experience of epilepsy can be very different from someone else's. Some seizures appear as unusual behaviour, such as staring, repeated swallowing or fluttering eyelids. Others cause loss of consciousness, although this can be so brief that nobody notices. And some seizures mean that people's muscles stiffen and jerk.[8]

Over the years, the way that doctors classify seizures has changed and in 2017, the International League Against Epilepsy published a new way of grouping and naming seizures.[9]

Not everyone with epilepsy has triggers, but certain things can increase the likelihood of a seizure in some people. Triggers vary between individuals, but can include not taking epilepsy medicine as prescribed, feeling tired or stressed, having an excess of alcohol or recreational drugs, flashing or flickering lights, missing meals or having a fever.

Epilepsy is a workplace issue

Common myths persist about what jobs you can and can't do if you have epilepsy, and some people think that epilepsy prevents you from doing certain jobs. In fact, people with epilepsy work in most jobs. Unless they have a good reason, employers shouldn't use your epilepsy as a reason not to give you a job. A 'good reason' could be if your epilepsy is a risk to your health and safety, or somebody else's, or because you don't have the relevant driving licence.

Rules about epilepsy and driving depend on what kind of seizures you have, when they happen and when you last had one, as well as the class of vehicle you want to drive.[10]

Under the Equality Act 2010, epilepsy may be considered as a disability if it has a substantially adverse and long-term effect on your ability to carry out normal day-to-day activities. The Act protects you from unlawful discrimination at all stages of the employment – from recruitment and employment conditions to dismissal and redundancy – and requires employers to make 'reasonable adjustments' (see box).

Supporting people with epilepsy at work

When you're offered a job, you are not obliged to tell your employer you have epilepsy provided it's well controlled and does not affect your ability to work safely and effectively. But if your epilepsy does affect your safety at work – and you have not told your employer – they may be able to dismiss you.[11]

There are, however, good reasons to talk to your employer about your epilepsy. It means they can make reasonable adjustments (see box). It also means that you comply with the Health and Safety at Work Act 1974, under which you are responsible for your own – and other people's – health and safety at work, and ensures you're covered by your employer's insurance. And it can be helpful to tell your colleagues about your epilepsy, because it will help them know how to help you if you have a seizure at work. Epilepsy Action publish guidance on first aid for different kinds of seizure.[12]

If you have epilepsy, your employer must carry out an individual risk assessment to ensure you can work safely. What the risk assessment covers depends on your job, but could include what type of seizures you have, how well they're controlled, any triggers, whether or not you get a warning before a seizure, and if you need any special care after a seizure.

If you might have a seizure at work, it's sensible to draw up a care plan with your employer. Based on the risk assessment and your experience, it could include how your colleagues can help you during and after a seizure, how you get home and who travels with you.

Ways that your employer could help you at work include working fixed hours rather than shift work, ensuring you don't work alone, altering triggers for disciplinary action for sickness absence and bonus targets, and having a disability leave policy that allows additional time off for medical appointments.

There are many other things that employers can do to make workplaces epilepsy-friendly, regardless of whether they need to make reasonable adjustments for an employee with epilepsy. Doing this proactively and collectively can help make workplaces better for everyone. The TUC has a useful list of actions that unions can ask an employer for, including a place to rest and relax, training for managers and staff about epilepsy, and epilepsy to be included in harassment and bullying policies.

Cancer is a workplace issue

More than 750,000 people of working age in the UK are living with cancer, and almost 120,000 people of working age are diagnosed with cancer each year. Thanks to better treatments, more people now survive. Together with an ageing population (see chapter 8), this means that employers will need to do more to support people with cancer at work.

After a cancer diagnosis, some people remain at work; others take time off during their treatment before returning to work, sometimes in a different role or with reduced hours; but some do not return to work. This may be a positive choice, but it can also be because they are not getting the support they need.

Research in the UK showed that one-fifth of people who returned to work after a cancer diagnosis said their employer and colleagues didn't understand their needs, and almost half were not entitled to sick pay, or had no access to flexible working or workplace adjustments. Other studies show that two to three years after a cancer diagnosis, only 64% of employees return to work successfully.[13]

These figures reveal that many employers need to do more to support workers with cancer, including those whose cancer is terminal. In 2016, the TUC launched a campaign called Dying to work. As well as seeing a change in the law, the campaign asks employers to sign a charter detailing how they will support employees with a terminal illness (see box).

There are other reasons why cancer is a workplace issue. If you have – or have had – cancer, you're legally protected from unfair treatment at work. The Equality Act 2010 makes it unlawful for an employer to discriminate against you because of your cancer. It also means employers should make 'reasonable adjustments' to help you stay at work or return to work (see box).

For many people, work and workplace colleagues are important sources of support during a period of huge uncertainty. And work is a crucial source of income at a time when outgoings can increase significantly. A 2013 survey by Macmillan Cancer Support found that for 83% of cancer patients, their illness cost them £570 a month in extra travel expenses, parking charges etc. Added to this, one-third of people lost £830 a month in pay because they were unable to work, or reduced their hours.[14]

How your employer can help

If you have been diagnosed with cancer, telling people about it can be very difficult; however, there are advantages to talking to your employer about your diagnosis. It means that they can make changes to your job or workplace that will help you work during treatment, or when you return to work afterwards. And if you have – or have had cancer – the law protects you against discrimination (see box).

The kind of support you need will depend on your cancer and your treatment. Side effects of treatment vary, but they can include feeling very tired and having no energy, being at greater risk of infection and bleeding, numbness in your hands and feet, and memory problems. Not everyone responds to the same treatment in the same way, so Macmillan Cancer Support suggests waiting until your first treatment before deciding what to do about your work. There are many adjustments that can help you stay at work, including changing your working hours or your duties.[15]

If you decide not to work during treatment, your employer should make adjustments to your job or workplace to enable you to return to work. Recent research by IOSH looked at how employers could best help people return to work after cancer, and identified several areas of good practice. These included: having a plan for returning to work; regular contact between employer, employee and colleagues before returning to work; building up hours gradually; and conducting individual risk assessments. Risk assessments should be followed up regularly because of the changeable nature of some long-term symptoms.[16]

Risk assessments should cover physical aspects of the job and take into account factors such as fatigue and pain, working hours and flexible working, as well as practical matters such as risk of infection, journey to work and parking facilities.

CASE STUDY   Dying to work

In 2016, the TUC launched a campaign to have terminal illness recognized as a 'protected characteristic' so that an employee with a terminal illness would enjoy a 'protected period' where they could not be dismissed as a result of their condition. The campaign, which began when Jacci Woodcook – a 59-year-old sales manager and union member – was forced out of her job after being diagnosed with terminal breast cancer, is called 'Dying to work'.[17]

As part of the campaign, the TUC is asking employers to sign a voluntary charter setting out an agreed way in which their employees will be supported, protected and guided throughout their employment, following a terminal diagnosis. Energy company E.ON was the first company to sign the charter in 2016 and when Royal Mail signed in 2017, it meant that more than half a million UK workers had these guaranteed rights in the event of being diagnosed with a terminal illness.

About diabetes

Around 3.5 million people in the UK have diabetes. Since 1996, the incidence of diabetes has more than doubled and estimates suggest that by 2025 there will be 5 million people with diabetes in the UK.

Diabetes is a serious, life-long health condition. It occurs when the amount of glucose in the blood is too high, which if untreated can cause serious health complications. There are two main types of diabetes, Type 1 and Type 2; these are different conditions with different causes.

Type 1 diabetes is an autoimmune condition where, because the body destroys its own insulin-producing cells, your body can't make insulin. Although type 1 diabetes can develop at any age, it's the most common form of diabetes in children. Overall, around 10% of people with diabetes have Type 1, and everyone with Type 1 is treated with insulin.

Type 2 diabetes happens when the body doesn't make enough insulin, or the insulin doesn't work correctly. It's caused by a mixture of genetics and environmental factors, and having a healthy lifestyle makes a big difference to reducing your risk of developing Type 2 diabetes.

Diabetes is a workplace issue

Although many people with diabetes do not consider themselves as having a disability, the Equality Act 2010 defines disability as a life-long condition which has a serious impact on your day-to-day life, which means that many people with diabetes are considered as having a disability under the Act – whether or not they would consider themselves disabled. The Act protects you from unlawful discrimination at all stages of the employment – from recruitment and employment conditions to dismissal and redundancy – and requires employers to make 'reasonable adjustments' (see box).

People with diabetes shouldn't be restricted in the jobs they can do because of their diabetes, and it is unlawful for employers to operate blanket bans on recruitment of people with diabetes. However, some jobs involving safety-critical work, such as the emergency services, have requirements that may be difficult for some people with certain medical conditions, including diabetes, to meet. Decisions about someone's suitability for these jobs should be based on an individual assessment and involve a medical adviser with experience of diabetes.

Shift work used to be seen as problematic for people with diabetes, but improvements in blood glucose testing mean it's less likely to be an issue.

Having diabetes doesn't mean that you can't drive – or do a job that involves driving. However, your treatment will make a difference to which vehicles you can drive, how often you must have your licence renewed, and what you need to tell the DVLA.[18]

Supporting people with diabetes at work

Many people manage their diabetes without it affecting their work. You should tell your employer that you have diabetes so that they can make reasonable adjustments. These might include adjusting your working hours, giving you time – and somewhere clean and private – to test your blood glucose levels and inject insulin, providing special equipment if you develop diabetes-related complications (such as visual impairments), and counting diabetes-related sickness absence separately so that it doesn't trigger disciplinary action.[19]

Information and support

There is a lot of information online about how to cope at work with eplilepsy, migraines, cancer or diabetes, and other conditions such as arthritis and asthma:

Arthritis Care www.arthritiscare.org.uk/living-with-arthritis/ working-with-arthritis

Arthritis Research UK Working with arthritis and joint pain www.arthritisresearchuk.org/arthritis-information/daily-life/ work-and-arthritis.aspx

Asthma UK Having asthma at work www.asthma.org.uk/advice/ living-with-asthma/work

NHS Advice for employees on working with a long-term medical condition www.nhs.uk/Livewell/workplacehealth/Documents/ ChronicConds_Employees_Factsheet_A4.pdf

National Migraine Centre www.nationalmigrainecentre.org.uk

Migraine Action www.migraine.org.uk

Migraine Trust www.migrainetrust.org

Macmillan Cancer Support tel: 0808 808 00 00

Fit For Work tel: 0800 032 6235 (English), 0800 032 6233 (Welsh), in Scotland 0800 019 2211

Epilepsy Action helpline tel: 0808 800 5050, www.epilepsy.org.uk

To find out more about epilepsy and driving, visit www.epilepsy. org.uk/info/driving

Notes

1 Macmillan Cancer Support (2013) Health and work service workshop for long-term conditions: Note of discussion. www.macmillan.org.uk/documents/getinvolved/campaigns/mps/finalreportofhealthandworkserviceworkshop.pdf)

2 Business Disability Forum Factsheet for employers on migraines. https://members.businessdisabilityforum.org.uk/media_manager/public/86/Resources/Factsheet%20on%20Migraines%2012_13.docx

3 Migraine Trust (2018) *Migraine: Help at work*. www.migrainetrust.org/wp-content/uploads/2018/02/The-Migraine-Trust-Help-at-work.pdf

4 National Migraine Centre Migraine triggers. www.nationalmigrainecentre.org.uk/migraine-and-headaches/migraine-and-headache-factsheets/migraine-triggers

5 Migraine Trust (2017) New poll fuels migraine work fears. www.migrainetrust.org/new-poll-fuels-migraine-work-fears

6 Migraine Trust (2018) *Migraine: Help at work*.

7 Equality Commission (2011) *Disability discrimination law in NI: a short guide*. www.equalityni.org/ECNI/media/ECNI/Publications/Individuals/DisabilityDiscrimShortGuide2011.pdf?ext=.pdf

8 TUC (2017) *Epilepsy in the workplace: a TUC guide*. www.tuc.org.uk/sites/default/files/EpilepsyInTheWorkplace.pdf

9 ILAE (2017) *New ILAE seizure classification*. www.ilae.org/news-and-media/news-about-ilae/new-ilae-seizure-classification

10 Epilepsy Action, *Work and epilepsy*, www.epilepsy.org.uk/sites/epilepsy/files/B135-Work-and-epilepsy.pdf

11 Ibid.

12 See www.epilepsy.org.uk/info/firstaid

13 IOSH (2017) *Return to work after cancer*. www.iosh.co.uk/returntowork

14 Macmillan Cancer Support (2013) *Cancer's hidden price tag.* www.macmillan.org.uk/Documents/AboutUs/Newsroom/ Cancers-Hidden-PriceTag-exec-summary-April-2013.doc

15 Macmillan Cancer Support. *Work and cancer.* www.macmillan. org.uk/information-and-support/organising/work-and-cancer

16 IOSH (2017) *Return to work after cancer.*

17 Dying to work: www.dyingtowork.co.uk

18 DVLA. *Diabetes and driving.* Available at www.gov.uk/diabetes-driving

19 See Diabetes UK (2015) *Employment and diabetes advocacy pack,* www.diabetes.org.uk/resources-s3/2017-09/Advocacy% 20pack_EmploymentV3-Jan2016_0.pdf and USDAW (2016), *Diabetes: An advice guide for USDAW reps.* www.usdaw.org.uk/ CMSPages/GetFile.aspx?guid=543fac95-42c2-4a6a-be38-71963898fc31

Chapter 16
Migrant workers

If you are a migrant worker in the UK, you are entitled to exactly the same health and safety protection as anyone else at work, even if you are not working in the UK legally. Depending on the type of work that you are doing, your health and safety will be enforced by either the Health and Safety Executive (HSE) or a local authority or council (see chapter 19). You may also come across the Gangmasters and Labour Abuse Authority (GLAA). The chances of an inspector visiting you to make sure things are satisfactory, however, are small, so it is vital that you are aware of your rights and how to make sure you are working healthily and safely.

Although this chapter is aimed at migrant workers, it is vital that other workers look out for the conditions in which their migrant colleagues are working and help them speak up and secure improvements. Experienced workers are usually best placed to spot risks, and unsafe and unhealthy conditions endanger everyone at the workplace, not just migrant workers. An employer that is prepared to exploit migrant workers is likely to be cutting corners elsewhere.

Why you may be at particular risk

A migrant worker is typically someone who has come to Britain from abroad to work within the previous five years and has been working here in the previous 12 months. Many migrant workers speak good English and have the same working conditions as non-migrant workers. They are often highly skilled but working in jobs with which they are not familiar or do not have the right skills. Poor English, vulnerable employment or residency status and low pay can increase the risks significantly, with migrant workers too often enduring long hours with little protection in illegal conditions and almost certainly without the benefit of trade union membership. The TUC has produced a guide for union safety representatives on migrant workers.[1]

The HSE highlights factors that may, as a migrant worker, place you at particular risk.[2] You may:

- have problems communicating in English, and therefore be less able to talk effectively with other workers and supervisors, particularly about your understanding of risk;

- be unfamiliar with workplace risks and have not done the type of work that you are now being asked to do, particularly if you have worked in Britain only for a short period;

- have limited knowledge of the British health and safety system, your health and safety rights and how to raise issues and find help;

- find yourself working in hazardous conditions, particularly if you want to earn as much as you can in as short a time as possible;

- have limited access to health and safety training and difficulty in understanding what is being offered; and

- be working in a situation where there are unclear responsibilities for health and safety, in particular where you are supplied by a recruitment agency or labour provider (which is the person or company that supplies you to a 'labour user'), or you are self-employed.

Migrant workers

Around one in 10 workers in the UK is from overseas. Although migrant workers are employed throughout the economy, certain sectors and geographical locations (particularly the southeast) employ large numbers. Some of these sectors have higher than average ill health and injury rates and/or present particular health hazards:

- agriculture and food processing – up to half of the seasonal agricultural workforce comes from overseas. Particular health risks and conditions include musculoskeletal disorders (MSDs), noise-induced hearing loss, sun and heat exposure, chemicals and dust;

- cleaning – workers are usually working on sites away from their employer and often outside of normal hours. They are usually managed by, and dependent upon, the cleaning contractor, rather than the host. MSDs are a particular risk, as are skin problems (dermatitis) from cleaning materials;

- construction – particular health risks include asbestos, dusts and MSDs. Figures from the Office for National Statistics indicated that in 2016, non-UK workers made up 11% of the construction workforce in the UK but over 50% in London.[3] Migrant workers accounted for 44% of building workers earning low wages, suggesting an over-representation of migrant workers in low-paid work;[4]

- health and social care – more than one in three medical staff come from overseas. Major problems include work-related stress, violence, dermatitis and MSDs. Migrant workers may be unfamiliar with equipment, procedures and clinical practices used in the UK. Communication is of particular importance, both with other workers and patients;

- catering, hospitality and hotels – hazards and problems here include long and anti-social hours, violence and harassment, slips and trips, cleaning chemicals and scalding; and

- food and drink manufacturing industries – health issues include MSDs caused by repetitive work on production lines, dermatitis, asthma (from flour dust, for example) and noise-induced hearing loss.

Help in different languages

To help you, the HSE's migrant workers website[5] offers advice in 16 languages, as well as in English, covering what you should expect your employer to do and what you have to do, alongside a list of organizations that you can contact for help. It also provides answers to common questions you might want to ask, including on clothes and equipment that help protect you ('personal protective equipment' or PPE), toilet and washing facilities, drinking water, first aid, training, language issues, home country qualifications, pregnancy, raising concerns, employment rights, whether your employer can charge for accommodation and unsafe rented accommodation.

The languages are: Polish, Russian, Punjabi, Chinese, Romanian, Urdu, Bengali, Portuguese, Turkish, Hindi, Lithuanian, Czech, Slovak, Kurdish, Albanian and Latvian. The website also links you to free translations[6] of three short HSE guides in 19 languages – the 16 above as well as Arabic, Gujarati and Welsh. Two of the guides offer essential health and safety information and a guide to basic health and safety law for all workers. The third is a pocket card aimed specifically at overseas workers in agriculture and food processing (although the information is applicable to all industries).[7] The TUC has produced a short online guide to working in the UK. It covers eight areas, including health and safety and hours of work, and is available in Arabic, Bangla, Gujarati, Hindi, Mandarin, Punjabi, Tagalog and Urdu.[8]

What should you do?

As an employee, you have the same legal duties as non-migrant workers and must:

- not put other people at risk because of your work;

- help your employer to reduce health and safety risks in the workplace;

- use any equipment in the way that you were trained;

- use properly anything that is supplied to keep you safe and healthy; and

- tell your employer in writing if you are pregnant, breastfeeding or have given birth within the previous six months. If there are risks to your heath and safety or that of your baby, your employer must try to remove the risk. If it cannot remove the risk it should adjust your working conditions and/or hours of work, offer you suitable alternative work (at the same rate of pay), or suspend you from work on paid leave.

Your employer, however, is responsible for ensuring your health and safety and owes you the same duties as does any other employer to its workers. Although it can be sometimes difficult to determine 'the employer' when a labour provider supplies workers to a business, the HSE is clear that 'business and the labour provider have a shared responsibility to protect their health and safety, regardless of which one is the employer.'[9] Both parties should also clarify and formalize in writing their respective responsibilities.[10]

The HSE advises you[11] to make sure your employer has insurance (it should display an Employers' Liability Compulsory Insurance certificate) and that it has told you about the risks that it has identified in its risk assessment and what it has done to protect you against them.

Make sure you understand

Your employer must ensure that you have the information, instruction and training that you need to do your job safely. You must have training before you start (which is called induction training) and training related to the job you are doing. The training can be provided by the person or organization that is using your labour or by the organization that has supplied you to do the work (including an agency, labour provider or gangmaster). It is particularly important that you do not operate machinery without training.

It is not, however, just a matter of being told what to do (see box). Make sure that you understand what you have been told, the risks you face, what the safety signs mean and what you should do so that you can work healthily and safely. If you are unsure, tell your supervisor.

CASE STUDY   Lenka Toperczer

Case study: Lenka Toperczer

The importance of language and understanding was exemplified in an accident that left an agency trainee without four fingers. On 8 October 2014, the trainee, Lenka Toperczer, a Polish-speaking Slovakian, was working at a rotary knife lathe for her employer, Cheshire Mouldings and Woodturnings, at its factory in St Helens,

Lancashire. While turning a piece of wood, her hand was pulled into the lathe, amputating three fingers on her right hand and one on her left hand.

The HSE's investigation found that the company had failed to provide proper guarding and had not planned the task. Ms Toperczer had only been at the site for a few weeks and had been trained to operate the knife by a colleague from the same agency. Her colleague had only used the machine seven times and had not trained anyone previously.

Imran Siddiqui, the HSE inspector who investigated the accident, said the case showed the importance 'of clear communication, in whatever form or language, to ensure issues regarding safety are understood'. Although Mrs Toperczer was unable to communicate well in English, the 'training for the machines was not delivered in such a way that full understanding of the procedure could be confirmed with operators whose first language was not English'.

Fining the company £0.3 million at Liverpool Crown Court on 20 November 2017, the Recorder of Liverpool, Judge Clement Goldstone, said it was 'highly pertinent' that Mrs Toperczer's trainer, a 'Pole with limited English', was asked by his manager, 'an Englishman with limited Polish', to carry out the training. Nor were there any instructions in Polish, even though the company employed several Polish-speaking workers.

If you have problems understanding English, your employer can help you by:

- providing information in your language (but making sure it uses a competent translator familiar with any technical terms);
- teaming you with an experienced worker who speaks your language;

- using another employee who speaks both your language and English to act as an interpreter;

- bringing in a professional interpreter for particular purposes, for example for training sessions;

- seeking help from local organizations, for example Citizens Advice that may have contacts with overseas worker communities;

- thinking about different and additional ways of communication, for example online visual material and DVDs, audio tapes in your language, and internationally recognized signs and symbols;

- using simple, clear English in training sessions;

- training supervisors in how to communicate clearly. The HSE reports that some construction employers use multi-lingual supervisors, and translate instructions, guidance and training materials into the first language for their workers.

You can get help with improving your English, for example by taking an ESOL (English for Speakers of Other Languages) course.[12] You may have to pay for some courses, but others can be free. Some unions offer courses and help (see box).

CASE STUDY   United for Education

In December 2017, the Unite union celebrated the 10th anniversary of its United Migrant Workers Education Programme.[13] The programme was developed by branches and members of the union representing cleaners, domestic workers, Chinese migrants and hotel and catering workers.

Unite claims the programme has benefited more than 7,000 workers from 25 nationalities 'to integrate into UK society by a combination of ESOL and other complementary courses, covering not just language skills, but also dance therapy and art'. The programme, which is delivered at weekends, also offers workshops on health and employment rights that are delivered by partner charities, and on information and communications technology.

Make sure you can always speak to an experienced supervisor and that you can understand each other. If you are worried about your health or safety, talk to your supervisor, manager or employer and also to your union safety representative if there is one. If you are still worried, you should contact the HSE (see chapter 19). You can do this without giving your name and the HSE will handle your complaint so that it cannot be traced back to you.

Things to know

You should not pay for any PPE and clothing that you need to do your job, such as a helmet, safety goggles or boots. This is a legal requirement. Your clothing should also be warm and waterproof if you are working outside, for example on a farm or on a construction site. Your employer is not allowed to ask you to give a 'refundable deposit' for PPE either (which it would in theory give back to you once you have finished your contract). Make sure, however, that you return your equipment when you leave the job, otherwise the cost might be deducted from your final wages.

You are entitled to toilet and washing facilities, with soap and towels, and drinking water. These are particularly important if you are working in remote, outdoor locations or premises with manual activities, such as labouring or planting and harvesting food, and construction. You should also be provided with somewhere clean to eat and drink during breaks, rest and changing facilities and somewhere to store clothes and change if you need to wear special clothing during your work.

There are also limits on how long you have to work, time off, rest breaks and paid annual leave (see chapter 9). You need to know where the first aid box is kept and who is in charge of first aid. Your employer should explain the procedures for first aid and emergencies to you, and it is vital that you are aware of these.

Even if you have certificates and qualifications from your home country, they are unlikely to be recognized in England for health and safety law. Your employer can see whether the UK will recognize your qualification as 'equivalent' to one from the UK by contacting the UK National Recognition Information Centre.[14] If not, you will probably have to undergo training and take a test, particularly if you are doing something like using a chainsaw. If you are working in construction, you should try to obtain a card under the Construction Skills Certification Scheme. An employer will accept the card as proof of your skills.[15]

Gangmasters and Labour Abuse Authority

If you have been supplied by a gangmaster to work in the agriculture, horticulture, shellfish gathering or associated processing and packaging industries, your gangmaster will need to be licensed and comply with eight standards.[16] One of the standards concerns your health and safety and covers similar requirements to those described above (who is responsible for your heath and safety, risk assessment, instruction and training, PPE, welfare facilities, first aid and accident investigation). The standard also sets out transport requirements covering vehicles and drivers, as well as additional detailed requirements for shellfish gathering (this is a particular concern because of the 2004 Morecambe Bay tragedy, in which 23 Chinese migrants drowned while picking cockles). A second standard covers working conditions; it includes the right to join a trade union, and covers rest breaks, working hours, annual holiday (see chapter 10) and discrimination.

In addition to licensing the specified sectors, the GLAA was given responsibility in 2016 for tackling labour abuse across the whole of the UK economy. You can download a leaflet on your employment rights in the same 20 languages as those offered by the HSE above.[17] The leaflet covers pay, sick pay, annual leave, working hours and health and safety. The GLAA will help you if you think you are:

- not being paid properly (including the national minimum wage and holiday pay);
- not allowed the correct time off or breaks;
- not given the equipment that you need to do your job;
- have concerns about your health, safety or welfare;
- being housed in unhygienic or unsafe accommodation;
- travelling to and from work in unsafe vehicles; or
- threatened with violence.

The GLAA, along with the police and other agencies, is also tackling 'modern slavery', which includes slavery, servitude, and forced or compulsory labour and human trafficking. If you think you or a colleague or friend might be a victim, you can follow advice from the government[18] or telephone one of the numbers in the 'further help' box.

Further help

There are a lot of resources online to help migrant workers with their rights, including:

Individual unions produce guidance for and about migrant workers. For example: www.unison.org.uk/get-help/ knowledge/vulnerable-workers/migrant-workers/

HSE (reporting a problem), tel: 0300 003 1647 or: webcommunities. hse.gov.uk/connect.ti/concernsform/ answerQuestionnaire?qid=594147

Gangmasters and Labour Abuse Authority – to report a problem, tel: 0800 432 0804 or submit a form at: www.gla.gov.uk/ report-issues/#site-header (the form is available in English, Bulgarian, Polish. Romania, Latvian, Lithuanian, Portuguese and Slovak)

Modern Slavery Helpline, tel: 08000 121700 or www.modernslavery.co.uk

Salvation Army Human Trafficking Helpline: 0300 303 8151

Citizens Advice, tel: 020 7833 2181 and www.citizensadvice.org.uk (England and Wales); tel: 0289 023 1120 and www. citizensadvice.co.uk (Northern Ireland); and 0131 550 1000 and www.cas.org.uk (Scotland)

Advisory, Conciliation and Arbitration Service (Acas) helpline – free advice and help on your employment rights, tel: 0300 123 1100 and www.acas.org.uk/index. aspx?articleid=1461

Crimestoppers – to provide information about a crime. You do not need to leave your name and your call cannot be traced, tel: 0800 555 111; and www.crimestoppers-uk.org

Hazards magazine: www.hazards.org/migrants

Migrants Rights Network: migrantsrights.org.uk. The organization
has produced a guide, *Know your rights. A guide for
migrants*, which includes a section on employment:
migrantsrights.org.uk/wp-content/uploads/2018/03/Hostile-
Environment-WEB-1.pdf

Notes

1 TUC (2007) *Safety and migrant workers. A practical guide for
safety representatives*, www.tuc.org.uk/sites/default/files/safetymw.
pdf

2 www.hse.gov.uk/toolbox/workers/migrant.htm and www.hse.gov.
uk/migrantworkers/industry.htm

3 Office for National Statistics, *International immigration and the
labour market, UK: 2016*, bit.ly/2jfYSZ8

4 Rolfe H and Hudson-Sharp N (2016) *The impact of free
movement on the labour market: case studies of hospitality, food
processing and construction*, National Institute of Economic and
Social Research, bit.ly/2w44DT6. Reported in *Focus on Labour
Exploitation (2018)*, 'Shaky Foundations. Labour exploitation in
London's construction sector', www.labourexploitation.org/sites/
default/files/publications/Shaky%20Foundations.pdf

5 www.hse.gov.uk/migrantworkers

6 www.hse.gov.uk/languages/index.htm

7 HSE (2008) *Working in the UK from overseas? Your heath and
safety at work in agriculture and food processing*, INDG410,
www.hse.gov.uk/pubns/indg410.pdf

8 TUC (2017) www.tuc.org.uk/research-analysis/reports/working-
uk-guide-your-rights

9 www.hse.gov.uk/migrantworkers/employer.htm

10 www.hse.gov.uk/migrantworkers/employer.htm

11 www.hse.gov.uk/migrantworkers/worker.htm

12 Government advice on how to find help with improving your maths, English and IT skills: www.gov.uk/improve-english-maths-it-skills

13 uniteumwep.blogspot.co.uk/p/about-us.html

14 UK National Recognition Information Centre: www.naric.org.uk/naric

15 Construction Skills Certification Scheme: www.cscs.uk.com

16 GLAA (2017) *Licensing standards*, www.gla.gov.uk/media/3180/licensing-standards-may-2012-reprinted-june-2017.pdf

17 GLAA (2018) *Workers' rights*, www.gla.gov.uk/media/3012/glaa-workers-rights-12pp-a7-english.pdf

18 HM government (2015) *Help for adult victims of modern slavery*, bit.ly/2jfuEp3

Chapter 17
Violence and abuse

Every year, at least one in a hundred workers will suffer an assault, threat or verbal abuse or violence while at work. Unlike most of the issues covered in this book, the main risk arises from members of the public. This does not, however, absolve your employer of its duties, which are the same as for any work-related hazard – that is, it must assess the risks, implement preventive and protective measures, and generally ensure your physical and mental health and safety. There are, however, steps that you should take too to help make yourself safe at work and to cope with the mental and physical consequences should you be so unfortunate as to suffer an attack.

One in 100

The most recent Crime Survey for England and Wales found that an estimated 1.3% of working adults experienced violence that was connected to their work or their workplace in 2016/17.[1] Of the 326,000 victims, 132,000 were assaulted and 204,000 were threatened or abused.

Victims are often involved in more than one incident of violence (42% of victims in 2016/17), which means that the number of incidents is higher than the number of victims. In 2016/17, for example, there were an estimated 642,000 incidents (269,000 assaults and 372,000 threats).

Of the violent incidents, 36% resulted in physical injuries, the majority of which involved minor bruising or a black eye. Strangers were the offenders in 55% of cases. Where offenders were known, they were most likely to be clients or a member of the public known through work. Colleagues accounted for fewer than one in 10 perpetrators. In short, one in two assaults, and one in three threats, come from clients or customers who you will already know. There are other reporting sources that similarly point to a high incidence of violence at work (see box).

The incidence of violence

The Labour Force Survey estimated[2] 41,000 non-fatal injuries to workers as a result of acts of physical violence at work, which accounted for around 7% of all non-fatal injuries and 8% (364,000) of all working days lost due to workplace injuries.[3]

In 2016/17, employers reported to the Health and Safety Executive (HSE) 4,941 injuries to employees – including two fatalities – that arose from a 'physical assault or act of violence' that resulted in more than seven days off work. This represented 7% of all reported workplace injuries, a similar percentage to that identified under the LFS.

Which jobs are the riskiest?

The Crime Survey for England and Wales updates data by occupation every two years, so the latest figures published in 2018 are from 2015/16. This showed that you are at the greatest risk of violence where you have contact with the public; police officers, fire service officers, prison service officers and police community support officers face a 9.6% chance of being assaulted or threatened at work, against a national average of 1.3%. Jobs with notably increased risks are:

- health care professionals (3.1%);
- health and social care specialists (3.4%)
- transport and mobile machine drivers (3.0%).

Other professions that experience consistently higher rates of violence are public transport workers, catering and hotel workers, benefits staff, teachers, shopworkers (see box) and managers and personnel officers. Workers who are least at risk include those in agriculture plant and storage-related occupations, science and technology professionals, and associate professionals and workers in administrative occupations.

Shopworkers

Violence is a particular problem in the retail sector, which employs one in 10 workers in the UK. The British Retail Consortium's latest Retail Crime Survey[4] found the rate of reported violence with injury in 2017 was six per 1,000 shopworkers, which was twice that of the previous year. Put another way, 13 shopworkers were injured in a violent incident every day of the year, including weekends. There were also 40 incidents of violence and abuse per 1,000 workers, which is the second highest level recorded, albeit lower than the previous year. Knives and other stabbing implements were the most significant weapons present in the incidents, followed by syringes.

The biggest concern, according to the BRC, comes from:

the growth in severe violent incidents against staff. BRC members report that career criminals intentionally use violence and abuse when challenged over stealing. The increasingly common requirements for retail colleagues to age-check and refuse sales, is also triggering increasing violence and threats.

A survey by the Association of Convenience Stores (ACS)[5] estimated that there were 13,437 violent incidents in convenience stores in 2017, of which 39% resulted in injury. There are around 50,000 stores in the UK. A weapon was used in 3,690 incidents (64% involved a knife, 17% a firearm and 19% 'other weapons' such as an axe, screwdriver or a hammer). Furthermore, 72% of staff experienced verbal abuse. The top three causes of aggressive behaviour were challenging shop thieves, enforcing an age-restricted sales policy and refusing to serve drunks.

The shopworkers' union, Usdaw, runs a regular survey as part of its Freedom From Fear campaign. This showed that in 2017, 62.34% of shopworkers were verbally abused (an increase of 25%), 40.49% were threatened (an increase of 38%) and there were 265 assaults each day (over 2%, and a 25% increase).[6] The 2016 survey found that of shopworkers who were abused, over 10% experience it at least weekly.

What can you do?

Before we look at what you can do, it is important to reiterate that your employer is required by law to ensure your health and safety, which includes preventing exposure to violent, abusive and threatening behaviour. This arises from the general duty of care that your employer owes you, as well as its duties under specific laws, notably to ensure your health and safety under the Health and Safety at Work Act 1974, and to carry out a risk assessment and implement preventive and protective measures under the Management of Health and Safety at Work Regulations 1999.

The HSE advises employers to adopt a four-step management process to control violence based on risk assessment; finding out whether there is a problem; determining who might be harmed and how; implementing an action programme including a safe system of work; and checking and monitoring the efficacy of the arrangements.[7]

You too have a duty to take reasonable care of your own health and safety and that of others. This means that you should adhere to your employer's policies and follow its procedures, take part in training that is offered to you, and report procedures that are problematic and any incidents of violence to your employer.

Planning ahead

The Suzy Lamplugh Trust recommends you always PLAN ahead:

- Prepare – think in advance about the 'what ifs'.
- Look confident – preparation will increase your confidence but, even if it does not, try to appear as if you are (without looking confrontational).
- Act to avoid risk the moment you become aware of it.
- Never assume that you will not be attacked or that your fears are unfounded. Instead, trust your instincts.[8]

Take every incident seriously, even if you were not hurt or troubled. Low-level aggression is often a harbinger of worse things, and a near miss may be a serious incident that has, by luck, not ended in injury. Near misses may also highlight an underlying trend or problem. List any work-related situations where you have felt at risk, and note down:

- what occurred and where;
- your reaction;
- whether the incident could reoccur and, if so, what you would do differently; and
- whether you told anyone and, if not, why not?

Even if you have not suffered violence, it is important to envisage what might go wrong. Try using the four Ws: who might commit violence; where might it occur; when might it occur; and what might you be doing?

Who: Think about the people you will meet in the course of your work. Potential perpetrators include customers, clients, the general public and even your colleagues. Do they have a history of violence? Are they likely to welcome your presence, and what you are meeting them about?

Where: Will you ever have to meet someone alone in a public or private space, such as a person's home? Is the location in a rural or isolated area?

When: Are you meeting the person during office hours, or early morning or late at night when your colleagues are not around?

What are you doing? Certain types of tasks may expose you to an increased risk of violence. Even among 'low-risk' occupations, there may be tasks that will nonetheless increase the risk of violence. The tasks below that may place you at increased risk are drawn from those highlighted by the Suzy Lamplugh Trust, the Health and Safety Executive, the National Health Service and individual trade unions. These tasks, of which more than one may well be present, include:

- handling money;
- providing health care to people who are ill, panicked or afraid of what might happen to them (especially in the NHS and ambulance services);
- confronting a suspected shoplifter or a customer who is attempting fraud, notably shop workers and security staff;
- dealing with difficult and unpredictable situations, as for example the police and fire services do;
- providing a security service, for example 'bouncers' and door staff, particularly where you might be refusing admission or searching for drugs;

- dealing with people who are angry or feel they have failed;

- meeting the friends and families of patients or clients who are anxious, angry, afraid or find it difficult to cope with the bureaucracy from which they are seeking help;

- where you are representing authority and enforcing rules or regulations, including council and HSE inspectors. (The Labour Party's 2017 general election manifesto promised it would 'consult on toughening the law against assaulting workers who have to enforce laws' and noted that they faced 'regular abuse'[9]);

- providing, or having the power to withdraw, an essential service or benefit, for example staff who are dealing with people who face a benefits cap or are helping people return to work;

- dealing with clients who are frustrated by what they perceive as poor services;

- carrying out repairs inside people's homes, for which they might not want to pay or feel aggrieved that the equipment has broken;

- selling alcohol (pubs and clubs);

- dealing with people under the influence of alcohol or drugs. (The 2016/17 Crime Survey for England and Wales found that workers who experienced a threat or physical assault considered the offender to be under the influence of alcohol in 36% of assaults and 25% of threats. The influence of drugs was present in 21% of assaults and 13% of threats);

- talking about sensitive matters;

- carrying medical drugs or supplies;

- when you are unable to help a client; and

- working with vulnerable and some mentally ill people.

Ask yourself

Below, we set out some specific questions that you should ask yourself as a matter of course. Do not wait until there has been a violent incident.

- Did your employer consult you when it was assessing the risks of violence, and did the assessment look at your job and the risks you face?

- Have you received training in agreed personal safety procedures and how to manage specific situations you may face?

- If you have to work alone for long periods without supervision, have you received specific training and are you satisfied with the arrangements?

- Have you been trained in dynamic risk assessment? (This allows you to assess risks as they arise and is particularly useful in a place with which you might not be familiar, for example when visiting a client's home.)

- Are you aware of how you report all incidents of violence, threats, abuse and near misses to an allocated line manager?

- Do you know what to do in an emergency and who to contact (and how)?

- Do you have a personal alarm or panic button that you know how to use, and are the devices tested regularly? (The Suzy Lamplugh Trust lists 22 lone worker apps and devices, although it does not endorse any particular product.[10])

- Have you received self-defence training? (You should, however, use this only as a last resort when other options are exhausted.)

- Do you report to your employer anything that you see as potentially problematic, or that might help avoid or diffuse a tricky situation? For example, if you see frequent queues near your workstation, are there sufficient refreshments, drinking water, toilet facilities, seating and information on queue times? (Although your employer should be checking all of these, if you are on the frontline you may be more aware of potential triggers.)

- If you have made a report or complaint, has it been treated appropriately?

- If you deal with members of the public, suppliers, clients and customers, are they able to see a notice displayed prominently by your employer stating that it has a zero tolerance policy to violence, that staff are supported and deserve respect, and that abuse will not be tolerated and prosecuted?

- Has your employer made a clear statement to its staff that violence will not be tolerated and will be treated as a disciplinary offence (including the possibility of dismissal or criminal action)?

- If you work with cash, is it kept out of sight?

- Do you have a safe or secure area to which public access is not possible?

- Are public car parks and access ways well lit?

- Has your employer deployed CCTV in public spaces? This can help reduce violence but should only be introduced after consultation with your representatives or you and your colleagues. Advice on CCTV good practice is available from the Information Commissioner[11] and the Home Office.[12]

Meeting strategies

If you are meeting a client or customer for the first time, try to avoid seeing them alone, or make sure a colleague is nearby, or meet where you are easily visible. If the meeting is in an office:

- sit near to the door, and between your client and the door, and have a strategy for exiting, for example you could say you need to go to the toilet, make a cup of tea or fetch some paperwork;

- have a pre-arranged code word for colleagues (similarly if you are receiving abuse while on the phone); and

- make sure you have rules for stopping an interaction should it start to pose a threat to you.

If you are visiting clients in their home by yourself, there is excellent advice available from the Suzy Lamplugh Trust[13] and the TUC, as well as individual unions. Broadly, you should:

- carry out your own 'dynamic' risk assessment when you approach the client's home' and again once you are inside. If you feel at all uncomfortable or unsure, make an excuse and leave;

- use a tracing system whereby you log in or alert a colleague as you are about to enter the home and as you leave. This should include the client's address and phone number;

- use a system that allows you easily to alert a colleague or your employer should you feel at risk;

- think about arranging for a colleague to ring you after an agreed number of minutes into a meeting, particularly with a new client, to check that you are safe and feel comfortable with them. Have a predetermined code word in case you need to summon help without alerting the client; and

- think about potential exit strategies should you feel uncomfortable or threatened. These should involve the location of the doors as well as an excuse for exiting the room.

People can become angry and aggressive when they are frustrated, frightened or unable to cope. When dealing with such people, remember to control your own tension (see box) and:

- make sure you have been trained in, and are confident in your use of, tactics for defusing a situation;
- avoid body language that might be perceived as aggressive, for example crossed arms or a raised arm;
- never place a hand on someone who is angry;
- respect personal space;
- never turn your back on an aggressor; and
- consider a diversion technique, for example shouting to people to call for the police.

How to control tension

The Suzy Lamplugh Trust advises that changes to the body when faced with tension, such as a racing heart, can be useful because they act as alerts. Many people, however, freeze when confronted or threatened, which led the trust to suggest you practice control techniques so that you can regain control of your reactions, think more clearly and make safer choices:
   While sitting in a chair:

- clench your hands into tight fists;
- release completely including your arms, shoulders, jaw and neck. Breathe out a sigh as you release;
- stretch your fingers out as far as you can;

- release as above;
- push your shoulders down. Release;
- push your back down into the chair. Release;
- push your heels into the floor. Release;
- expel all breath as a sigh so that your lungs fill with air;
- slowly breathe in one long breath, filling your lungs;
- expel again as a sigh; and
- repeat as often as you can.[14]

If you have suffered violence

If you have suffered an abusive or violent incident at work, you should talk to someone. This can be a friend or a colleague but you must also talk to your union or safety representative, if you have one, and also to your line manager or supervisor. Do not remain quiet because of any feelings of sympathy you might have if, for example, your assailant was desperate because of benefit problems or worried about their health. A person who resorts to violence once is likely to do so again and a failure to report the incident puts you and your colleagues at risk in the future from the same assailant. Also, if you do not report a problem, your employer might not be aware of it and so cannot improve security. Later, you should make sure that your employer has reviewed and improved its arrangements for preventing violence and abuse so that you and your colleagues are not placed at a similar risk. Remember too that inspectors from your local authority or the HSE may investigate the incident, with the police usually involved in the more serious incidents.

If you have suffered violence, you may have sustained a physical injury, which will be obvious and treated by a first aider at work, your GP or hospital. Less immediately obvious, but potentially more damaging, are mental traumas. You may feel one or more of:

- anxious, panicky, jumpy or tense;
- not wanting to leave the house or go to work;
- angry or irritable;
- numb;
- restless;
- emotional or tearful;
- powerless or worthless;
- confused;
- depressed or down;
- other symptoms of stress;
- tired; and
- alone or isolated.

It is common too to suffer flashbacks or nightmares and suffer problems with sex, concentrating, eating or sleeping. These should diminish after a week or two but if they do not, or they appear later, you should visit your GP. One of the conditions for which your GP will look is post-traumatic stress disorder, which commonly involves:

- reliving details of the event in nightmares or the belief that it is occurring again;
- avoiding doing anything that reminds you of the incident;
- increased irritability, sleep disturbance, outbursts of anger and sudden shock reactions.

You may need counselling to help you come to terms with what you have been through. This will be available through your employer's employee assistance programme or occupational health service (see chapter 12). If your employer does not have either provision, your GP will put you in touch with a counselling service.

Your employer should also provide you with support and consider making temporary or permanent adjustments to the way you work, for example if you were attacked while working a late shift, you may prefer to work during the daytime only. You may also need some time away from your job.

You may be able to claim compensation from your employer with a civil claim (see chapter 19) or to make a personal injury claim to the Criminal Injuries Compensation Authority (CICA)[15]. This must be for a medically recognized physical or mental condition that has been caused by an act of violence, or by attempting to prevent an offence, which has been reported to the police. You have two years from the date of the incident in which to make a claim; any award will reflect the extent of your injuries, loss of earnings and needs such as care.

Further information

There is a good deal of online information about how to deal with violence or potential violence in the workplace:

Health and Safety Executive: www.hse.gov.uk/violence/

National Institute for Health and Care Excellence (2015); Violence and aggression: Short-term management in mental health, health and community settings, NICE guideline, www.nice.org.uk/guidance/NG10

The Suzy Lamplugh Trust (advice on personal safety): www.suzylamplugh.org; tel: 0808 802 0300

Victim Support, the national charity providing support to victims of crime: www.victimsupport.org.uk; or the Victim Support line: tel: 0808 1689 111 or via a police station

Victims' Information Service (Home Office): www.victimsinformationservice.org.uk

USDAW (advice on violence in the retail sector): 'Freedom from Fear' campaign: www.usdaw.org.uk/Campaigns/Freedom-From-Fear

UNISON (2013): *'It's not part of the job: a health and safety guide on tackling violence at work'*, www.unison.org.uk/content/uploads/2013/07/On-line-Catalogue216963.pdf

GMB union advice for security staff: www.gmb-security.org.uk

RMT (train workers): 'Charter of protection against violence', www.rmt.org.uk/news/public-document-library/transport-workers-charter-of-protection/

National Education Union (2016), 'Violence and assaults against staff in schools: model policy for employers', (also contains model reporting form), www.teachers.org.uk/help-and-advice/health-and-safety/v/violence-and-assaults-against-staff-schools

Notes

1 HSE (2018) *Violence at Work, 2016/17. Findings from the Crime Survey for England and Wales and from RIDDOR*, www.hse.gov.uk/statistics/causinj/violence/index.htm

2 Labour Force Survey statistics: www.hse.gov.uk/statistics/lfs/

3 HSE (2018) *Violence at Work, 2016/17*

4 BRC (2018) *2017 retail crime survey*, brc.org.uk/media/249703/2017-crime-survey-short-story_fa_63_v11.pdf

5 Association of Convenience Stores (2018). *The crime report 2018*, bit.ly/2H4mwmF

6 www.usdaw.org.uk/About-Us/News/2017/Nov/Violence-threats-and-abuse-against-shopworkers-is

7 HSE (2006) *Violence at work. A guide for employers*, INDG69, www.hse.gov.uk/violence/HSE

8 Suzy Lamplugh Trust (2017) *Personal safety at work: a guide for everyone*, www.suzylamplugh.org/Handlers/Download. ashx?IDMF=04509d26-fd53-40dc-9413-8c1aa42e0b8c

9 *For the many. Not the few.* The Labour Party manifesto 2017. bit. ly/2reg3zN

10 www.suzylamplugh.org/Pages/Category/lone-worker-directory

11 Information Commissioner (2015) *In the picture. A data protection code of practice for surveillance cameras and personal information*, ico.org.uk/media/1542/cctv-code-of-practice.pdf

12 Home Office (2013) *Surveillance camera code of practice*, assets. publishing.service.gov.uk/government/uploads/system/uploads/ attachment_data/file/282774/SurveillanceCameraCodePractice.pdf

13 Suzy Lamplugh Trust (2017) *Personal safety at work: lone working*, www.suzylamplugh.org/Handlers/Download. ashx?IDMF=61d3260c-818f-4646-8b3e-e2f09d1152a7 and www.suzylamplugh.org/FAQs/lone-working

14 Suzy Lamplugh Trust (2017) *Personal safety at work: a guide for everyone*.

15 CICA advice line: 0300 003 3601. CICA advice on making a claim: www.gov.uk/government/organisations/criminal-injuries-compensation-authority

Chapter 18
Gender and transgender issues

Everyone has an equal right to protection from harm at work. But this equality of protection does not mean that every worker is the same, or is exposed to the same hazards. This chapter explores the idea of gender-sensitive health at work and focuses on the occupational health needs of trans people, women who are pregnant, breastfeeding or going through the menopause.

Gender and health at work

Gender has clear influences on workplace health, so it's vital to integrate gender in occupational health to create healthy workplaces for everyone. Since the late 1990s, researchers, trade unions and occupational health professionals have begun to pay more attention to occupational health and women workers.[1] Developments in health and safety law, policy and risk management were primarily based on work traditionally done by men, and research on workplace health often ignored work traditionally done by women.[2] As a result, women's workplace health was largely ignored, under-diagnosed, under-reported and under-compensated.[3] Today, unions and employers' groups are also beginning to focus on trans workers, who are often at higher risk of bullying, harassment and abuse at work (see chapters 3 and 17).

Gender impacts workplace health in many ways. Some of these come from the physical, physiological and psychological differences between men and women. Others arise from their different employment experiences. And a third influence stems from the fact that women and men have different responsibilities outside the workplace. Women form 46% of the UK workforce, but there is still strong occupational segregation in the labour market, both in terms of sector and seniority. This means that women and men may be exposed to different hazards at work.[4]

A simple example of this is the way that personal protective equipment, tools and workstations were designed and set up in the past. Having been traditionally designed with men in mind, PPE was often uncomfortable or a poor fit for women, as well as for some men. Ignoring gender reinforces these problems, so trade unions have long argued for a 'gender-sensitive' approach to health at work – one that acknowledges these differences so that everyone's health can be protected.[5]

The Canadian Centre for Occupational Health and Safety provides a range of information, research and resources on gender, work and health,[6] and the TUC publishes a useful gender checklist on occupational safety and health, encouraging trade union reps to bring together equalities work with workplace health.[7]

Transgender health at work

We've seen that creating safe, healthy and supportive workplaces means acknowledging gender differences and taking a gender-sensitive approach to health at work. For transgender workers, this means acknowledging the fact that the workplace can be a daunting environment for some. Transgender or trans is often used an umbrella term for a multitude of gender identities. Some people may identify as transgender, some as transsexual and others as non-binary, so trans embraces individuals with many different experiences, needs and wishes.

As far as health at work is concerned, it's important for employers and trade union representatives to be aware of legislation, policies and practicalities related to transgender issues in the workplace. Creating inclusive and supportive working environments also clearly depends on how we all act, talk and think about gender.[8] It's also important to be aware of the scale of discrimination. Surveys show that 60% of trans workers have experienced discrimination at work, more than half feel that they have to hide their gender identity from colleagues, and 88% say that ignorance remains the greatest challenge they face at work.[9]

Trans workers still face distinct challenges at work, including gendered facilities, discrimination, bullying and harassment (see chapter 3). One in eight trans employees were physically attacked by a colleague or customer during the past year, according to a survey by Stonewall, which publishes a range of information for trans employees and advice for employers on creating inclusive workplace environments.[10]

For trans people at work, the *Transgender workplace support guide* offers 10 top tips for trans employees. Because of the importance of having strong allies at work, the guide's number one piece of advice is to think about who you would like to share your gender identity with. The list also includes talking to your employer; what your personal timeline looks like if you want to come out at work – and whether this means you need time off; looking up your employer's policies on discrimination, absence and harassment; finding out about legislation and where to get support.[11]

As well as the law on workplace health (see chapter 19), there are other pieces of legislation that protect trans employees. The Equality Act 2010, which promotes equality and protects people from unfair treatment, includes gender reassignment as a 'protected characteristic'. This means it's unlawful to discriminate against someone, or treat them unfairly, because of gender reassignment. The Act defines gender reassignment broadly: it covers you if you are undergoing, have undergone or are proposing to undergo gender reassignment, and it uses a personal – rather than a medical – definition of gender reassignment. For some people, transition involves medical assessments and treatment. The Act means it's unlawful for employers to treat these absences less favourably than absence due to illness or injury. The Gender Recognition Act 2004 covers people who want to legally change their gender from that stated on their birth certificate.[12]

Employers should have policies that cover the support they offer transitioning workers as well as practical issues such as dress codes, toilet facilities, personal records and communication. It's good practice for employers to take a generous and flexible approach to absence for health and other appointments for staff during transition. Managers should talk to employees about the help and support they would like during transition; people in customer-facing jobs might prefer temporary adjustments such as home working or a back-office role while transitioning, for example.[13]

Pregnancy

Two pieces of health and safety legislation – the Management of Health and Safety at Work Regulations 1999 (MHSW) and the Workplace (Health, Safety and Welfare) Regulations 1992 (the Workplace Regulations) – include specific requirements for new and expectant mothers at work. Under MHSW, your employer's risk assessments should include any specific risks to new and expectant mothers and women who could become pregnant, including:

- physical hazards, such as vibration or radiation, manual handling;
- biological and chemical hazards, such as exposure to infectious diseases, cytotoxic drugs, carbon monoxide, lead and mercury;

- stress;

- working hours;

- travel; and

- temperature.

Employers must regularly review risk assessments, which includes any changes in risks associated with different stages of pregnancy. This is important, because unborn babies may be at greater risk earlier and later in pregnancy.

The law says that if risks cannot be removed, your employer must temporarily adjust your working conditions or your hours. If this isn't possible, then you must be offered 'suitable alternative work' at the same pay or, if this cannot be done, then your employer must suspend you and give you paid leave. We've seen in the chapter on shift work that working nights can adversely affect your health. If your GP or midwife thinks that your night shifts will affect your health, they can give you a certificate to take to work. Your employer must then offer you suitable alternative work at the same pay or, if this isn't possible, they must suspend you and give you paid leave.

The Workplace Regulations specifically cover the facilities that employers must provide for pregnant or breastfeeding workers, including somewhere for you to rest and lie down. It's also good practice, the HSE says, for employers to make sure you have somewhere safe to express milk and store it (although this isn't a specific legal requirement). And although you don't have to tell your employer that you are pregnant, breastfeeding or have recently given birth, it's important to do this so that they can make sure you are protected from hazards at work. Until you inform them in writing, your employer isn't required to adjust your working conditions or hours of work.[14]

If you need more help and advice, speak to your occupational health service (see chapter 12) or trade union representative.

Menopause

The menopause affects all women, but has been largely ignored as a workplace issue. In 2015, the UK's Chief Medical Officer Professor Dame Sally Davies challenged the taboo that still surrounds talking about the menopause at work. 'I want to encourage managers to ensure working women feel as comfortable as possible discussing menopausal symptoms as they would any other issues affecting them in the workplace,' she said.

There are many reasons why the menopause is a workplace issue. Women make up 46% of the UK workforce and because the workforce is ageing (see Chapter 8), the menopause affects an increasingly large number of women at work.[15]

Women's experiences of the menopause vary widely. Although three-quarters of women in the UK seek advice about their symptoms – which can include hot flushes, night sweats, tiredness, memory problems, low mood, irritability and aching limbs – most say they aren't much trouble. However, 20–25% of women say that their hot flushes and night sweats adversely affect their work and quality of life, primarily because they cause sleep loss, fatigue and affect concentration.

CASE STUDY   Menopause at work: A personal story

I am a part-time self-employed swimming teacher and also do freelance work building websites for small businesses and charities. For me, the menopause is all about loss: loss of certainty, of status, of confidence. My short-term memory is poor, so I check and double-check things anxiously. I feel I can no longer rely on my brain.

It's also happening in a period of my life where I have lost a parent, am having to consider the needs of the other parent and my son is starting his GCSEs. I have had a recurrence of severe depression and feel that this has been exacerbated and prolonged by the menopause. It is the first time in my life I have had suicidal feelings. So whether or not some of these feelings have been as a result of the menopause, they have certainly been intensified by the menopause. And it's the first time that I have thought maybe I will never recover again.

I have hot flushes which are disconcerting and uncomfortable. Luckily they don't affect me severely and working in a swimming pool is actually a very soothing experience.

To manage the symptoms I am seeing a CBT therapist, I take anti-depressants, I am going to start HRT to see if it helps. Being able to work part-time rather than full-time helps. And having a rewarding and non-stressful job.

Work has been my salvation as it has helped me keep structure in my life and forced me to keep going. It is a part-time job so it has given me lots of opportunity to rest and I could not have maintained it on a full-time basis. My employers are very supportive but I have no job contract so if I were not able to stick to my schedule I would not be paid and would eventually be replaced. The job is very rewarding and not too demanding so it's quite like having occupational therapy. However, I still feel extremely anxious at times about it and have thought I wouldn't be able to keep doing it.

I have mentioned menopausal symptoms to my colleagues and my employer but not in a particularly serious way. I work mainly with women who also happen to be a lot younger than me. One woman mentioned that her Mum was going through it too. It's hard to know how they would react, I think they would be kind but there would be nothing in place if a woman needed any adjustments.[16]

Many employers have been slow to recognize that women of menopausal age may need special consideration. A TUC survey of 500 safety representatives found that 45% said their managers did not recognize problems associated with the menopause, and that the working environment was making menopausal symptoms worse. Two-thirds of safety reps said that warm workplaces caused problems for menopausal women, and half said workplace stress made things worse.[17]

It's estimated that 10% of women have taken days off work because of menopausal symptoms and 10% of women stop work altogether because of their severe symptoms.[18] And recent research – the first large-scale survey of women's experience of working through menopausal transition in the UK – found that one third of women felt their performance at work was negatively affected by menopausal symptoms and 53% said it was difficult to manage work during the menopause.[19]

Despite this, it seems that few women feel comfortable talking to managers about the menopause. A survey of teachers by the NUT found that 80% did not want to raise symptoms with their employer because they were embarrassed or afraid of being targeted by management.[20]

Tackling the taboo

Employers can do a lot to support women going through the menopause. What women need will depend on their own experience, but when researchers asked women which workplace changes were most helpful, the following were mentioned most often: management awareness of menopause as a possible health problem; flexible working hours; information and advice from employers about menopause and coping at work; better temperature control and ventilation; and access to informal support at work.[21]

Including information on the menopause in workplace wellbeing policies, sharing this with the wider workforce and providing training for managers can all help encourage more open discussion. Henpicked – an online community of 'women who weren't born yesterday' – has advice on how to have confident conversations with your manager.[22]

CASE STUDY Menopause policies – University of
Leicester

In 2017, the University of Leicester became the first UK university to
introduce a workplace menopause policy to enable staff to have
confident conversations around menopause and show leadership on
the issue.[23]

The University also holds a popular 'Menopause: Let's talk about
it' workshop and a 'Menopause roadshow' – a series of one-hour
events across campus to allow staff to find out more about the
policy and start discussing the menopause more openly – and in
2018, launched its new 'Menopause Café', a free and informal
monthly meeting to chat about menopause matters. Menopause Café
was set up in Perth, Scotland in 2017 and the idea is spreading
around the UK.[24]

Tackling stress at work is also important. Stress can trigger hot
flushes and women aged 45–55 report high levels of work-related
stress, according to the Labour Force Survey (see chapter 2).

Policies on flexible working should recognize and support
women going through the menopause. Some women might find
it helpful to change their usual working practices, so offering
flexible working, different shift patterns or later start times can
help. Sickness absence policies should cater for menopause-
related sickness absence, and Business in the Community recommends that menopause-related sickness absences should be
recorded as an ongoing health issue rather than a series of short
term absences.[25]

Notes

1 Messing K (1998) *One-eyed Science: Occupational health and women workers*, Temple University Press, Philadelphia

2 WHO (2006) *Gender equality, work & health*. www.who.int/gender/documents/Genderworkhealth.pdf

3 TUC (2017) *Gender in occupational health and safety*. www.tuc.org.uk/sites/default/files/GenderHS2017.pdf

4 UNISON (2016) *Gender, safety and health: A guide for UNISON safety reps*. www.unison.org.uk/content/uploads/2016/07/23965.pdf; BITC (2012). *Women and work: The facts*. https://gender.bitc.org.uk/all-resources/factsheets/women-and-work-facts

5 TUC (2017) *Gender in occupational health and safety*. www.tuc.org.uk/sites/default/files/GenderHS2017.pdf
TUC (2017) *Personal protective equipment and women*. www.tuc.org.uk/sites/default/files/PPEandwomenguidance.pdf

6 CCOHS Gender, work and health portal: www.ccohs.ca/genderhealth/

7 TUC (2017) *Gender checklist on occupational safety and health*. www.tuc.org.uk/research-analysis/reports/gender-checklist-occupational-safety-and-health

8 Transgender Workplace Support Project (2016) *Transgender Workplace Support Guide*. www.lgbthealth.org.uk/wp-content/uploads/2016/07/TWSP-Info-Guide-Final.pdf

9 TUC (2016) *Transforming the workplace*. www.tuc.org.uk/sites/default/files/Transformingtheworkplace.pdf

10 Stonewall (2018) www.stonewall.org.uk/news/new-research-exposes-profound-discrimination-trans-people-face

11 Transgender Workplace Support Project (2016) *Transgender Workplace Support Guide*.

12 Acas. *Gender reassignment*, www.acas.org.uk/index.aspx?articleid=2064; Unison (2015). *Transgender workers rights*. www.unison.org.uk/content/uploads/2015/05/TowebTransgender-workers-rights.pdf

13 Acas (2017) *Supporting trans employees in the workplace.* www.acas.org.uk/media/pdf/6/f/Supporting-trans-employees-in-the-workplace.pdf; Department of Health (2008). *Trans: A practical guide for the NHS.* www.ncuh.nhs.uk/about-us/equality-and-diversity/documents/transgender-nhs-guide.pdf

14 HSE (2013) *INDG373: New and expectant mothers who work.* www.hse.gov.uk/mothers/index.htm

15 Department of Health (2015) *The health of the 51%: women.* www.gov.uk/government/uploads/system/uploads/attachment_data/file/595439/CMO_annual_report_2014.pdf. Department for Education (2017) The effects of menopause transition on women's economic participation in the UK. www.gov.uk/government/uploads/system/uploads/attachment_data/file/632403/menopause_report.docx

16 Anonymous.

17 TUC (2013) *Supporting women through the menopause.* www.tuc.org.uk/sites/default/files/TUC_menopause_0.pdf

18 Newson, LR (2018) *Menopause and work.* https://menopausedoctor.co.uk/what-is-the-menopause/menopause-work-new-guidelines

19 Griffiths, A, MacLennan, SJ and Hassard, J (2013) 'Menopause at work: an electronic survey of employees' attitudes in the UK', *Maturitas,* **76,** pp. 155–159. www.maturitas.org/article/S0378-5122(13)00223-5/pdf

20 NUT (2015) *Teachers working through the menopause.* www.teachers.org.uk/files/menopause-a4-for-web--9968-.pdf

21 Griffiths A et al. (2013) 'Menopause at work'. Faculty of Occupational Medicine (2017) Guidance on menopause and the workplace. www.fom.ac.uk/health-at-work-2/information-for-employers/dealing-with-health-problems-in-the-workplace/advice-on-the-menopause

22 Henpicked (2017) *Menopause: how to have confident conversations with your manager.* https://henpicked.net/menopause-how-to-have-confident-conversations-with-your-manager

23 University of Leicester menopause policy: www2.le.ac.uk/offices/ hr/docs/policies/menopause-policy-guidance

24 Menopause Café model: www.menopausecafe.net

25 Business in the Community (2017) *Women, menopause and the workplace.* https://age.bitc.org.uk/sites/default/files/women_ menopause_workplace.pdf

Chapter 19
Realizing your rights

This book has looked at what you can do to help ensure your health at work. Later in this chapter, we look at what you can do should things go wrong. It is important, however, to have a basic understanding of the UK's health and safety system and of your employer's legal duties and responsibilities within that system. Essentially there are three tiers to the legislation:

1 Underpinning the whole of the system is the Health and Safety at Work Act 1974,[1] which places general duties on employers and others, and sets out the UK's health and safety regulatory system, including inspections, enforcement, offences and penalties, union-appointed safety representatives (see box), and the making of secondary legislation (specific Regulations).

2 The Management of Health and Safety at Work Regulations 1999 set out the core requirements to carry out a risk assessment and implement preventive and protective measures.

3 There are then more than 100 sets of Regulations that are usually issued under the HSW Act and that address specific hazards, issues, groups of workers, industries or types of work, including display screen equipment, manual handling, use of work equipment, the workplace, personal protective equipment, major accident hazards, hazardous substances, asbestos, lead, noise and first aid at work. We have covered these Regulations where appropriate in previous chapters.

Union safety representatives

A trade union can appoint health and safety representatives at workplaces where the union is recognized. The representative has a legal right to: represent employees in discussions with the employer on health, safety or welfare and in discussions with the HSE or other enforcing authorities; investigate hazards, dangerous occurrences and complaints; inspect the workplace and relevant documents; attend safety committees; and to receive their normal salary (paid time off) for time spent on carrying out their functions and to undergo training.

There is conclusive evidence that trade unions and trade union-appointed safety representatives significantly improve workplace health and safety standards.

Much of the evidence is reviewed in two TUC publications,[2] among the highlights of which are:

- a 1995 study, and a 2004 follow-up, using data from the 1990 Workplace Industrial Relations Survey, that found that British manufacturers with health and safety committees had an injury rate that was half that of non-unionized manufacturers; and

- a 2007 report from the Department of Trade and Industry (DTI) that found safety representatives saved society between £181 million and £578 million a year by reducing the days lost from work-related injuries and illnesses by between 286,000 and 616,000 days. The TUC subsequently updated the figures to show that the benefits to the economy in 2014 of the contribution of union representatives to workplace injuries and ill health were between £219 million and £725 million.

The HSE has consistently highlighted the benefits of representation and worker participation in health and safety. For example, in 2015 guidance, it stated: 'Evidence shows that businesses with good workforce involvement in health and safety perform better in health and safety measures, and also tend to have better productivity and higher levels of workforce motivation.'[3]

The general duties

The HSW Act places general goal-setting duties on:

- employers to ensure the health, safety and welfare of their employees, particularly in relation to the provision and maintenance of plant and systems of work, dangerous and hazardous substances and articles, the workplace (including getting in and out of the workplace), the working environment, and the provision of information, instruction, supervision and training to employees;

- employers to conduct their undertakings so that they do not expose non-employees to risks, including contractors, clients, visitors, patients in hospitals, residents in care homes and members of the public. A similar duty applies to some self-employed workers;

- persons who have any degree of control of premises to ensure that the premises (including the entrances and exits), and any plant or substance that is present, are safe and without risk to health;

- designers, manufacturers, importers or suppliers of 'articles' (equipment) that are used for work to ensure that they are safe and without risk to health; and

- employees to take reasonable care of the health and safety of themselves and others who might be affected by the actions they take or choose not to take, and to cooperate with their employer to enable it to perform its duties.

The risk assessment

The Management of Health and Safety at Work Regulations 1999[4] provide the bedrock of health and safety management. They require employers to carry out a suitable and sufficient risk assessment covering employees and non-employees, the purpose of which is to identify what it needs to do to comply with its statutory health and safety duties. HSE guidance[5] depicts risk assessment as a five-step process in which the employer: identifies hazards; decides who may be harmed; evaluates the risks and decides on precautions; records the significant findings; and reviews and, if necessary, updates, the risk assessment. The risk assessment must cover physical and psychosocial hazards.

The HSE is explicit that when carrying out a risk assessment, an employer should consult its employees and health and safety representatives because it is 'a valuable way of involving the staff who do the work. They know the risks involved and scope for potentially dangerous shortcuts and problems. Employees are more likely to understand why procedures are put in place to control risks and follow them if they have been involved in developing health and safety practices in their workplace.'[6] This does not, however, mean that you need to be formally consulted before every task-specific assessment. The HSE is also clear that employers should check with its employees whether the risk assessment has missed anything.

Protect and survive

After carrying out a risk assessment, the MHSW Regulations require your employer to:

- implement preventive and protective measures following nine principles of prevention, starting with avoiding risk but, where this is not possible, a hierarchy of control measures;

- introduce arrangements for the planning, organization, control, monitoring and review of the preventive and protective measures;

- ensure the provision of health surveillance where appropriate;

- appoint one or more competent persons to help it comply with its health and safety duties;

- provide employees with information on the risks and the preventive measures and training; and

- implement specific measures in relation to young workers and new and expectant mothers (see chapters 14 and 18)

The MHSW Regulations require you, as an employee, to:

- use machinery, equipment, dangerous substances, transport equipment, means of production or safety devices provided to you by your employer in accordance with any training and instruction you have received; and

- inform your employer, or any employee responsible for health and safety, of any work situation you reasonably consider a serious and immediate danger and of any shortcomings in your employer's protection arrangements for health and safety in so far as they relate to your own work.

Solving a health and safety problem

If you have a health, safety or wellbeing issue, you should raise it with your employer, usually via your line manager or supervisor. As we note above, you have a legal duty to do this. You should also raise it with your union health and safety representative or shop steward, if you have one. It is always better to solve the issue before you or a colleague is hurt. If you are addressing a health and safety issue at a disciplinary or grievance hearing, you have the right to request you are accompanied by a union officer, a lay union official or shop steward, or a colleague.

If your employer fails to address the issue adequately, you can contact the enforcing body for your workplace. With a small number of exceptions, this will be either the HSE or one of 380 local authorities (see box). If you are raising an issue with the HSE, you should either fill out an online form or ring a central number.[7] The HSE will assess within 24 hours whether it will look into your complaint and, if it does take it up, will telephone, write to or visit your employer. It will also tell you within 21 days what action it is taking. If your workplace is enforced by the local authority, you should telephone or email its environmental health department (or equivalent); the details will be on the local authority's website.

Which body enforces health and safety at your workplace?

The HSE enforce health and safety at:

- factories;
- construction sites;
- central and local government premises;
- schools and colleges;
- hospitals and nursing homes;
- major accident hazards sites;
- offshore installations;
- gas, electricity and water systems;
- farms;
- mines;
- fairgrounds.

Local authorities enforce health and safety at:

- offices (except government offices);
- shops;
- hotels;
- restaurants;
- leisure premises;
- sheltered accommodation and care homes;
- nurseries and playgroups;
- pubs and clubs;
- privately owned museums;
- places of worship.

Other bodies responsible for health and safety at work enforcement cover:

- nuclear installations – Office for Nuclear Regulation;[8]
- railways – Office of Rail and Road;[9]
- flight and cabin crew – Civil Aviation Authority;[10]
- marine – Maritime and Coastguard Agency.[11]

Join a union

The best advice we can give you is to join a union, and to join before you have a problem at work. There are well over 60 unions in the UK with members in every job and profession, from football and music to health, finance, hospitality, manufacturing and all the public services. There will be a union that is right for your job. The TUC's website lists them all, or you can use the TUC's union finder at tuc.org.uk/join-union. If you are a member of a union that your employer recognizes, you have a far greater chance of a quicker and better outcome because your representative and employer will be well versed in using formal and informal procedures to resolve matters. The benefits of union membership will obviously stretch well beyond your physical and mental health too, although improvements in pay and conditions and representation can all link to health.

If your employer does not recognize the union of which you are a member, you should seek advice from your union, which can also supply a union officer to accompany you in formal meetings. If your workplace has a union, but you are not a member, you should join. Although the union may not help you with a problem that existed before you joined, it might be able to offer some help. It might also do so in a non-unionized workplace as it may allow it to recruit new members. While most unions require a minimum period of membership before offering legal representation, a local branch may well be able to provide advice and support around issues such as occupational sick pay and the employer's absence management procedures. In addition, if local union representatives become aware of management failings, they may be able to intervene to ensure that you and your colleagues are not injured in future.

In the sections below, we look at some of the ways in which you might secure compensation or benefit should you suffer harm. Again, you will have a far greater chance of success in claims against your employer (and its insurer) if you are a union member. The TUC has published a helpful and comprehensive guide, *Your Rights at Work*, which includes a section on enforcing your rights.[12] Whatever you do, you will need to collect evidence immediately, particularly if you intend pursuing a claim for damages. The evidence you will need includes: a note of how the incident occurred (date, time and place); the injury or illness; record of accident book entry; plans and photographs of the workspace and equipment; full contact details for witnesses; a diary of symptoms, medical treatment and absence; receipts for all expenses related to the incident; and payslips.

Employment tribunal

Some health and safety-related issues are handled in the Employment Tribunal, particularly those involving working time, discrimination, whistleblowing (Public Interest Disclosure Act 1998) and unfair dismissal. You usually have three months in which to bring a claim. Legal help is only available for discrimination claims brought under the Equality Act 2010. The average awards are in the single thousands of pounds. If your employer does not pay an Employment Tribunal award, you can now submit a Penalty Enforcement Form.[13]

Industrial Injuries Disablement Benefit

You might be entitled to Industrial Injuries Disablement Benefit (IIDB)[14] under the Industrial Injuries Scheme if you became ill or disabled as a result of an accident in the course of your work, or if you suffer from one of more than 70 'prescribed' diseases or conditions.[15] You must have been employed, or on been on an approved employment training scheme or course, in England, Scotland or Wales at the time of the accident. You cannot apply for IIDB if you were self-employed.

Unlike making a personal injury claim against your employer (see below), IIDB is paid on a no-fault basis, so you do not have to prove your employer was negligent. You should apply for IIDB no earlier than two months after your accident, and as soon as possible after you know you have a prescribed disease. With two exceptions, you will need to be assessed as at least 14% disabled. (The starting points for deafness and pneumoconiosis – lung disease caused by inhalation of dust – are 20% and at 1% respectively.) As examples, the assessments of disability are:

- 100% for diffuse mesothelioma (a type of cancer caused by asbestos), loss of both hands, absolute deafness, and loss of sight such that you cannot perform any work for which eyesight is essential;

- 30% for loss of vision in one eye;
- 20% for loss of two fingers on one hand; and
- 14% for loss of index finger or great toe (3% for any other toe).

IIDB is in theory payable for most injuries arising from a work-related accident providing you meet the disability conditions.

Payments for the 70-plus prescribed diseases (see box) are often restricted to specified industries, occupations or jobs (for example osteoarthritis of the hip in farm workers) and some require you to have worked for a specified number of years. You have to show that you have a prescribed disease and worked in one of the occupations specified for the disease (if applicable), but you do not have to prove a causal link. The prescribed diseases list excludes some of the most common work-related ill-health conditions, particularly many musculoskeletal disorders and stress-related illnesses. It is possible, though, to claim for some health conditions – for example, a back injury – if they were the result of an accident.[16]

Prescribed diseases

The 70-plus prescribed diseases that qualify for Industrial Injuries Disablement Benefit include:

- asthma;
- carpal tunnel syndrome;
- chronic obstructive pulmonary disease (a collective term for a range of lung diseases, including emphysema and chronic bronchitis);
- deafness;
- dermatitis (inflamed or irritated skin);

- diffuse mesothelioma and a number of other asbestos-related diseases such as primary carcinoma of the lung, pneumoconiosis (asbestosis) and unilateral or bilateral diffuse pleural thickening;

- pneumoconiosis (including silicosis and asbestosis);

- vibration white finger, which is a secondary form of Raynaud's disease caused by prolonged use of vibrating tools or machinery. Raynaud's disease is characterized by poor blood circulation in the extremities such as your hands and feet.

What will you receive?

The table below shows the weekly tax-free IIDB payment that you will receive depending on the assessment of the percentage of your disability. The rates are valid until April 2019. Payments range from £34.96 for an assessment of 14%–24% to £174.80 for 95%–100%.

TABLE 19.1 Industrial injuries disablement benefit: what might you be entitled to?

Assessment of disability	Percentage of IIDB payable	Weekly IIDB payment at 2018/19 rates
14%–24%	20%	£34.96
25%–34%	30%	£52.44
35%–44%	40%	£69.92
45%–54%	50%	£87.40
55%–64%	60%	£104.88
65%–74%	70%	£122.36
75%–84%	80%	£139.84
85%–94%	90%	£157.32
95%–100%	100%	£174.80

Compiled from: Department for Work and Pensions (2017), *Industrial Injuries Disablement Benefits: Technical guidance*; and Focus on Disability (2018), *Benefit rates in the UK for 2018 to 2019*, www.focusondisability.org.uk/brates-2.html

Receipt of IIDB can, however, affect many other benefits that you or your partner might be receiving, including Income Support, Housing Benefit and Universal Credit. If you are in receipt of IIDB, you can still make a personal injury claim, although any award may be reduced by the amount of your IIDB.

Some employers have their own separate compensation schemes, notably the Civil Service Injury Benefit Scheme[17] and the NHS Injury Allowance.[18] There are also government schemes for people with certain lung diseases including mesothelioma,[19] pneumoconiosis and byssinosis, in cases where the employer has gone out of business or cannot be traced.

Personal injury claims

If you suffer a personal injury that is caused or made worse by your work, you may be entitled to claim compensation from your employer (or its insurer). A personal injury encompasses disease, impairment of physical or mental condition, and death (in the latter case, your partner or family would obviously pursue the claim). The compensation will cover: pain, suffering and loss of quality of life (general damages); and loss of earnings and other financial losses, including the costs of adapting your home, future care needs and expenses (special damages). You may also be able to recover interest on the damages and some of your legal costs, but it is important to remember that, even where you win, government changes in 2013 mean that some of the costs of the case may be taken from your compensation awarded to you. Note too that most settlements are a few thousand pounds; the six and seven figures sums that you might read about in the media are rare and arise only where the future costs of care and loss of earnings are lengthy and substantial.[20]

For a claim to be successful, you must have suffered an injury that was caused by your employer's breach of its duty of care to you, and that it was foreseeable that the failure would lead to your injury. You must start proceedings within three years of the incident that led to your injury or from when you first realized you suffer from a disease or condition. This date is generally earlier than when a doctor will give you a confirmed diagnosis.

Most claims are settled out of court but if you do go to trial, your claim will be heard in the county court if it does not exceed £50,000, although if it is for a larger amount, it might go to the High Court.[21] If the claim for pain and suffering is no more than £1,000, the case will go to the small claims court, although no legal costs are recoverable here as the expectation is that there should not be legal representation. The Employment Tribunal can award compensation in a small number of specified instances, for example if you have suffered mental ill health as a result of a circumstance (usually discrimination or harassment) covered by the Equality Act.

It can be very expensive and time consuming to bring a case, regardless of whether your employer settles out of court or goes to trial, so in the first instance it is vital that you take good legal advice. If you are a union member, you should first approach your shop steward. Alternatively, you can contact your union's local office or its legal department. Initial contact details will be on your union membership card and the union's website. You will probably have to fill in a questionnaire and supply supporting evidence. Your union will likely retain the services of a firm of solicitors who are experts in employment rights. The solicitors will decide whether it is worth proceeding with your case. The decision will be largely based on your chances of success, but the solicitors or union may want to take up a less clear-cut case if it involves a new or interesting issue. The criteria can vary between unions. Crucially, if the union and its solicitors agree to take your case, it will not cost you anything.

If you are not a union member, or your union decides not to pursue your case but you wish to proceed, you will not receive legal aid. You should find out whether there is any good free or inexpensive legal advice available to you. Check whether any of your insurance policies covers legal expenses, free legal advice or representation. Contact some of the organizations listed in the 'free advice' box.

At some point, you will need to find a solicitor. Look for a member of the Association of Personal Injury Lawyers[22] or a solicitor with the Law Society's Personal Injury Accreditation.[23] Do not go to a firm of solicitors just because you have seen it advertising on television or online, and do not respond to 'cold calls'. The Law Societies of England and Wales, Scotland and Northern Ireland each have an online tool to help you search for a solicitor by category (including accident and injury, and employment) and by location.[24]

You might also want to consider engaging a solicitor on a 'no win, no fee' arrangement, in which the solicitor receives an agreed percentage – typically 25% – of any award but nothing if the claim is unsuccessful. This obviously reduces your financial liability but your compensation will be reduced too and there may also still be some initial costs as well as experts' fees. Such an arrangement may not be suitable if you have a particularly strong case that will result in a large payout. You will in any case need to consider taking out legal expenses insurance to pay your employer's costs should your claim fail – either because the judge finds against you or if the award is less than the amount your employer had offered as an out-of-court settlement.

You can often secure an initial meeting or telephone consultation with a solicitor free of charge and without obligation. After the meeting, the solicitor should inform you in writing of your chances of success, the likely compensation, the total legal costs and the terms on which the firm will take your case.

Free advice

A number af resources are available where you can get free advice on your rights in the workplace:

TUC online union finder: tuc.org.uk/join-union

TUC advice on personal injury claims: tuc.org.uk and search for 'personal injury claim'.

The Hazards Campaign is an influential UK-wide network of resource centres and campaigners with links to international networks such as the European Work Hazards Network, the Asian Network for Occupational and Environmental Victims and the National Council for Occupational Safety and Health in USA. It supports union safety representatives, individuals and groups fighting for the prevention of work-related diseases and injuries, and justice for those who have suffered. This includes challenging the victimization and blacklisting of union safety representatives and activists, and supporting and advocating for bereaved relatives through Families Against Corporate Killers. The campaign runs the annual grassroots Hazards Conference, a weekend of speakers, meetings and workshops attended by around 400 union safety representatives and activists. It also presses for improvements to policy, law and practice around health, safety and compensation issues, and works closely with *Hazards Magazine* (see below): www.hazardscampaign.org.uk; tel: 0161 636 7558; email: info@hazardscampaign.org.uk

Hazards Magazine is a quarterly publication produced by Rory O'Neill for union representatives, activists and workers on campaigning for and improving workplace health and safety. The magazine's website offers excellent information and advice on most of the issues covered in this book: www.hazards.org/index.htm

Citizens Advice, which was formerly known as Citizens Advice Bureau, is a network of over 300 independent charities that offer advice on a range of issues, including employment. Your local Citizens Advice may be able to put you in touch with a specialist lawyer: www.citizensadvice.org.uk/work/health-and-safety-at-work/accidents-at-work-overview

Law centres can offer legal advice, casework and representation to individuals who cannot afford a lawyer: www.lawcentres. org.uk/i-am-looking-for-advice. Check with the Law Centres Network to see if there is a centre that covers the area where you live: www.lawcentres.org.uk/about-law-centres/law-centres-on-google-maps/alphabetically

The LawWorks Clinics Network provides free initial advice to individuals on various areas including employment law. It operates in England and Wales and will put you in touch with volunteer lawyers, if you are not eligible for legal aid and cannot afford to pay for legal help. To find a clinic near you: www.lawworks.org.uk/legal-advice-individuals/find-legal-advice-clinic-near-you

AdviceUK has 700 members and advises a further 500 organizations. Although it will not advise you directly, you can use its website to find your nearest advice centre: www.adviceuk.org.uk/looking-for-advice/find-advice/

Public Concern at Work (PCAW) offer a confidential advice line that is managed by qualified lawyers with expertise in whistleblowing issues. PCAW operates as a legal advice centre designated by the Solicitors Regulation Authority. It advises on situations where others are at risk and will not advise directly on private employment matters: www.pcaw.co.uk; tel: 020 7404 6609

Acas Helpline: 0300 123 1100

Employment Tribunal Service: www.gov.uk/courts-tribunals/employment-tribunal. Enquiry Line: 0300 123 1024 (England and Wales) or 0141 354 8574 (Scotland).

The Equality Advisory Support Service (EASS) provides advice on discrimination issues and legal rights and remedies: bit. ly/2vHVGyo; tel: 0808 800 0082.

Notes

1 Health and Safety at Work Act 1974: www.legislation.gov.uk/ ukpga/1974/37

2 TUC (2016) *The union effect. How unions make a difference on health and safety*, www.tuc.org.uk/sites/default/files/ Unioneffect2015.pdf and TUC (2016), *The benefits of paid time off for trade union representatives*, www.tuc.org.uk/sites/default/ files/Facility_Time_Report_2016_0.pdf

3 HSE (2015) *Involving your workforce in health and safety*, HSG263, www.hse.gov.uk/pubns/priced/hsg263.pdf

4 The Management of Health and Safety at Work Regulations 1999, SI 1999 No. 3242. www.legislation.gov.uk/uksi/1999/3242/ pdfs/uksi_19993242_en.pdf

5 HSE guidance on risk assessment and links to free downloads: www.hse.gov.uk/risk/controlling-risks.htm

6 See also HSE (2015) *Involving your workforce in health and safety*, www.hse.gov.uk/pubns/priced/hsg263.pdf

7 Online form for reporting a health and safety problem to the HSE: webcommunities.hse.gov.uk/connect.ti/concernsform/ answerQuestionnaire?qid=594147. Alternatively, you can telephone: 0300 003 1647

8 www.onr.org.uk

9 www.orr.gov.uk/rail/health-and-safety

10 www.caa.co.uk/Safety-initiatives-and-resources

11 www.gov.uk/government/organisations/maritime-and-coastguard-agency/about/access-and-opening

12 TUC (2016) *Your Rights at Work*, fifth edition, Kogan Page

13 Details and form: www.gov.uk/government/publications/employment-tribunal-penalty-enforcement

14 IIDB: www.gov.uk/industrial-injuries-disablement-benefit

15 Department for Work and Pensions (2017) *Industrial Injuries Disablement Benefits: technical guidance*, www.gov.uk/government/publications/industrial-injuries-disablement-benefits-technical-guidance/industrial-injuries-disablement-benefits-technical-guidance

16 TUC (2016) *IIDB: a guide to claiming*. bit.ly/2FdXgri

17 www.civilservicepensionscheme.org.uk/media/181629/csibs.pdf and www.civilservicepensionscheme.org.uk/media/30019/ibs_feb2013.pdf

18 NHS Staff Council (2016). *NHS Injury Allowance – a guide for staff*, bit.ly/2HMMTQM

19 www.mesoscheme.org.uk

20 Extensive advice on personal injury claims is available at the TUC's website tuc.org.uk

21 Government advice on how to make a personal injury claim: www.justice.gov.uk/courts/procedure-rules/civil/rules/part07/pd_part07a

22 APIL, tel: 0115 943 5400. You can access APIL members who specialize in claims for work-related injures, and their accreditations, by location at: www.apil.org.uk/injury-lawyers/accident-at-work-lawyer

23 www.lawsociety.org.uk/support-services/accreditation/personal-injury

24 solicitors.lawsociety.org.uk; www.lawscot.org.uk/find-a-solicitor; and www.lawsoc-ni.org/solicitors

Index